SOUL MIND BODY
MEDICINE

SOUL MIND BODY
MEDICINE

A Complete Soul Healing System
for Optimum Health and Vitality

Dr. Zhi Gang Sha

New World Library
Novato, California

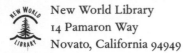

New World Library
14 Pamaron Way
Novato, California 94949

Text design and typography by Tona Pearce Myers

Library of Congress Cataloging-in-Publication Data
Sha, Zhi Gang.
  Soul mind body medicine : a complete soul healing system for optimum health and vitality / Zhi Gang Sha.— 1st ed.
    p. cm.
Includes index.
ISBN-13: 978-1-57731-528-5 (pbk. : alk. paper)
ISBN-10: 1-57731-528-6
  1. Holistic medicine. 2. Medicine, Chinese. 3. Mind and body. 4. Health.
  5. Vitality. I. Title.
R733.S492 2006
615.5—dc22   2005033907

First printing, May 2006
ISBN-13: 978-1-57731-528-5
ISBN-10: 1-57731-528-6

Printed in Canada on partially recycled, acid-free paper
Distributed by Publishers Group West

10 9 8 7 6 5 4 3

This book is dedicated to my most beloved and honored master, Dr. Zhi Chen Guo, Mama Guo, and their daughters. I am extremely honored to be Master Guo's worldwide representative and adopted son. Without his and his family's teachings, I could not have written this book. I cannot honor and appreciate them enough.

This book is also dedicated to my spiritual fathers in Jiu Tian (the nine layers of Heaven) and in Tian Wai Tian (the Heaven beyond Jiu Tian). I could not have written this book without their nourishment and blessing. I cannot honor them enough.

I also dedicate this book to the Divine. I am extremely honored to be a universal healer, teacher, and servant to spread divine teaching, healing, and blessing. I cannot honor the Divine enough.

Finally, I dedicate this book to all who are searching for the wisdom, knowledge, and practice of energy and spiritual healing, including the millions of people suffering from chronic pain, other chronic conditions, and life-threatening illnesses. You all need more help. This book is a practical tool giving you and your loved ones the help you need by teaching you how to heal yourselves and others.

I offer my love to everyone on Mother Earth and to every soul in the universe. Let me be your unconditional servant. My wish is for you to receive great benefits from the teachings of this book. I am extremely honored to serve you.

Thank you. Thank you. Thank you.

Contents

Chapter 3. Mind Over Matter....39

Chapter 4. One-Minute Healing....51

Chapter 5. Universal Meditation....67

Chapter 6. Applications of
Soul Mind Body Medicine....117

Chapter 7. Using the Four Power Techniques to Heal Common Ailments....175

Chapter 8. Preventive Maintenance....301

Chapter 9. The Essence....327

Preface

I have three missions. My first life mission is to teach healing, empowering people to heal themselves and others. My message for healing is:

I have the power to heal myself.
You have the power to heal yourself.
Together, we have the power to heal the world.

My second life mission is to teach soul wisdom, empowering people to enlighten themselves. The purpose of teaching soul wisdom is to help others fulfill their spiritual journeys, which consists of reaching soul enlightenment and further increasing one's standing in the soul world. My message for the soul journey is:

I have the power to enlighten myself.
You have the power to enlighten yourself.
Together, we have the power to enlighten the world.

My third life mission is to offer universal service. I am a universal servant. You are a universal servant. Everyone and everything is a universal servant. A universal servant offers universal service, which includes universal love, universal forgiveness, universal peace, universal healing, universal blessing, universal harmony, and universal enlightenment. My message for universal service is:

I offer universal service unconditionally.
You offer universal service unconditionally.
Together, we serve the universe unconditionally.

With Soul Mind Body Medicine, I have created a breakthrough healing system as a vehicle to carry all three of my life missions forward. This book will teach you how to heal yourself and others. It will also teach you how to do group healing and remote or distant healing. Furthermore, it will help you totally transform your soul, mind, and body. I am honored to present Soul Mind Body Medicine to the world.

My own healing journey has progressed for more than forty years, through study, self-development, clinical practice, teaching, and personal experience. I began studying tai chi at age six and qi gong at ten, and then quickly turned to the profound wisdom of kung fu, the I Ching, and feng shui. I studied Western medicine, receiving my MD in China. I also studied traditional Chinese medicine and became an herbalist and acupuncturist.

From my most respected master, Dr. Zhi Chen Guo, I learned Zhi Neng medicine (Zhi Neng means "the intelligence and capabilities of the mind and soul"). Much of the wisdom of Soul Mind Body Medicine comes directly from Master Guo's teachings. Without them, I could not have written this book.

As both an MD and a doctor of traditional Chinese medicine, I completely honor Western medicine, traditional Chinese medicine, and all other healing modalities. To create Soul Mind Body Medicine, I have synthesized the healing wisdom and knowledge of Western medicine, traditional Chinese medicine, Zhi Neng medicine, and Body Space Medicine, which I also learned from Master Guo, together with the spiritual healing knowledge gleaned from ancient philosophies and religions, including Buddhism, Taoism, Confucianism, and Christianity, as well as from many complementary and alternative healing modalities. I have also gained incredible wisdom and knowledge through my open spiritual channels, including my capabilities as a medical intuitive. After a lifetime of integrating all these studies and, finally, with guidance from Master Guo, my spiritual fathers in Heaven, my own soul, and the Divine (the Creator, the Source, or the universe), I have been able to develop Soul Mind Body Medicine.

My main purpose in writing this book is to create a road map for what I believe will be the future direction of medicine. At the same time, I strive to give you practical tools that will empower you to heal yourself and others, right away. You can learn Soul Mind Body Medicine without any medical or healthcare background.

I offer an approach to healing compatible with Western medicine and other healing modalities. This approach produces no adverse effects of any kind. It empowers you to assume a significant role in healing yourself and will assist you in restoring your health as quickly as possible. I hope that Soul Mind Body Medicine will lead you to think in a completely different way about medicine, health, healing, and life-transformation.

Many powerful healing techniques are revealed in the pages that follow. Each gem of wisdom is a powerful healing tool and a universal servant for your healing needs. Use each one with love, honor, and respect and it will bring immeasurable healing and blessings into your life.

Remember that unconditional universal service, including love and forgiveness, is the golden key that will unlock the gate of health for you, your loved ones, and the entire universe.

May *Soul Mind Body Medicine* serve you and others well.

Thank you. Thank you. Thank you.

Introduction

Over the past few decades, various forms of mind-body medicine have become more and more popular, to the point of being widely accepted. These modalities emphasize the mind-body connection, which encompasses the effects of our psychological and emotional states on our physical well-being and the power of conscious intent, relaxation, meditation, belief, expectation, and *mind over matter* to affect our health. Research in mind-body medicine is exploding. Physicians and hospitals are supporting, and in many cases even offering, mind-body practices, and health insurers are covering more of this treatment.

As both a Western- and Eastern-trained medical practitioner, I think mind-body medicine is a step forward, but it is not enough. It neglects the most important factor, the *soul*. The soul has consciousness, intelligence, and creativity. It also has power to heal and bless. Not only your own soul (your body's soul), but also the souls of your systems, your organs, and your very cells have the power to heal themselves and to heal you. In fact, we can communicate with the souls of our body, systems, organs, and cells, and ask them to heal themselves.

Since it is based on an understanding of the power of the soul, Soul Mind Body Medicine will be the breakthrough medicine for the twenty-first century. It emphasizes *soul over matter* as a complement to and major enhancement of *mind over matter*. Soul healing is the key to Soul Mind Body Medicine, and the origin of its fundamental principle: *Heal the soul first; then healing of the mind and body will follow.*

As we learn to heal ourselves through the power of the soul, communicating with the souls of our body, systems, organs, and cells and asking them to heal themselves, we can invoke all the Buddhas, saints, healing angels, ascended masters, and the Divine (whichever entities fit with your belief system) directly to request their healing and blessings. People understand how to invoke the spiritual world to heal through prayer, but the results they receive vary greatly. The reason is that one must follow certain spiritual principles and laws to receive maximum healing benefits from the spiritual world. In this book I will teach you this profound wisdom and reveal practical treasures for its application.

Practical treasures are the essence of *Soul Mind Body Medicine*. Many of these techniques have been carefully guarded since the time of the Yellow Emperor, five thousand years ago. They have been proven to work by tens of millions of people in China. In this book, you will find healing programs and prevention programs to restore and optimize your health, improve the quality of your life, and help you prolong your life.

Soul Mind Body Medicine's healing techniques work on the soul and the consciousness of the body's systems, organs, and cells. These techniques directly and instantaneously influence matter inside the cells and energy outside the cells. They also work on the emotional body to heal emotional imbalances like depression, anxiety, fear, anger, and grief. They work on the mental body to heal mental imbalances such as delusions and confusion. Finally, they work on the spiritual body, giving you techniques for clearing bad karma.

This book advances a unique theory, the Matter Energy Message Theory, to explain the cause of illness. It states that there are *three* main causes of ill health: matter blockages, energy blockages, and message or spiritual blockages. Matter blockages happen inside the cells. Energy blockages happen between the cells. Spiritual blockages happen in the Message Center, or heart chakra, and are due to bad karma, the sum total of mistakes one has made in this and previous lifetimes.

The techniques of Soul Mind Body Medicine work by recognizing the effects of message or spiritual blockages. Matter and energy are carriers of message. Message is soul or spirit; it communicates with and influences matter and energy. If you apply Soul Mind Body Medicine healing, the interplay between matter inside the cells and energy outside the cells will be adjusted and balanced immediately. This is how the soul or message works to offer healing. It is also why prayer works as a healing agent and why *soul over matter* is the heart of Soul Mind Body Medicine.

The real power behind *soul over matter* is unconditional love, forgiveness, and service. These are the golden keys to healing. *Love melts all blockages. Forgiveness brings peace. Everyone and everything is a universal servant.* In order to dissolve blockages and create healing, we apply unconditional love and forgiveness, along with the Four Power Techniques (Body Power, Soul Power, Sound Power, and Mind Power). Not only are these techniques simple, practical, powerful, and effective, but they are also easy to learn.

In this book I offer seven major methods for healing yourself and others:

1. *Say Hello Healing.* This technique invokes the power of the soul to heal. It is the key to Soul Mind Body Medicine and one of the simplest and deepest healing techniques you will ever learn. You can use Say Hello Healing to request healing from the inner souls of your body, organs, and cells as well as from the outer souls of holy beings and the souls of nature.

2. *Universal Meditation.* Universal Meditation invokes the healing power of the soul and mind of everything, from

the strands of your DNA to the sweep of the galaxies. With Universal Meditation, you can visualize any image in your own abdomen to nourish, heal, bless, manifest, and transform your life.

3. *The Golden Keys to Healing*. Love melts all blockages. Forgiveness brings peace. Service is the purpose of life. Use these golden keys to unlock the doors to health and the gates of life.

4. *One-Minute Healing*. One-Minute Healing is a quick and practical technique for removing matter, energy, and spiritual blockages. Use it anywhere, anytime, and every day to maintain your health.

5. *Four Power Techniques for Common Illnesses*. The Four Power Techniques are Body Power, Soul Power, Sound Power, and Mind Power. In this book, you will learn how to apply them to heal more than one hundred common health conditions.

6. *Healing Programs*. Consult this book for step-by-step protocols to restore your health if you are interested in boosting your energy, losing weight, reducing stress, balancing your emotions, or recovering from cancer.

7. *Prevention Program*. Healing is important, but prevention is vital. As the Yellow Emperor said more than five thousand years ago: *The best doctor is one who teaches people how to prevent sickness, not one who treats sickness.*

This book teaches time-honored practices that you can apply in less than thirty minutes a day to optimize your health, boost the quality of your life, and prolong your life. The techniques are simple and practical. You can learn them right away and apply them instantly for healing. You may receive significant results after a few applications, in a few days or in a few weeks. For serious, chronic, or life-threatening conditions, it may take several weeks or months to receive significant healing results and to restore your health completely. Soul Mind Body Medicine has already transformed many lives. It works.

⸎⸏⸎

Soul Mind Body Medicine is an unconditional universal servant, dedicated to healing you, your loved ones, your friends, and all humanity. It is also dedicated to serving every soul in the universe. It reveals profound healing techniques. It emphasizes unconditional love and forgiveness, the golden keys to healing. It guides you to realize that the purpose of life is to serve. It leads each soul to accomplish its destiny, which is to increase its spiritual standing. The final goal for every soul, on Mother Earth and in the universe, is to join as one to harmonize Heaven, Earth, and human beings.

Since healing is not limited to human beings, neither is Soul Mind Body Medicine. The practical tools of this medicine can be applied to your pets, plants, organizations, society, cities, countries, Mother Earth, other planets, other galaxies, and the entire universe. Ancient spiritual philosophy states, "A human being is a small universe. All of nature is a big universe. What happens in the small universe will happen in the big universe. What happens in the big universe will happen in the small universe." Soul Mind Body Medicine teaches you how to heal the small universe of a human being and the big universe of all of nature.

I am an unconditional servant to every human being on Mother Earth and every soul in the universe. Open your heart and soul to receive my love and service. I am honored and dedicated to serve you.

> *I love my heart and soul.*
> *I love all humanity.*
> *Join hearts and souls together.*
> *Love, peace, and harmony.*
> *Love, peace, and harmony.*

CHAPTER 1

Concepts of
Soul Mind Body Medicine

In this chapter, I explain the basics of Soul Mind Body Medicine, including its key theories, its diagnostic approach, and the fundamentals of healing. After reading this chapter, you will understand the key causes of sickness and how to heal from it. The rest of the book will give you a full toolbox of Soul Mind Body Medicine healing methods, including specific applications for many illnesses and guidelines for preventive maintenance.

Before exploring the basic theories of Soul Mind Body Medicine, let's first take a look at some of the fundamental concepts on which the theories rest, starting with the basis of the soul's healing power, and then the relationship between physical life and spiritual life.

SOUL POWER

The body and its immune system possess great healing potential. When you cut your finger, the cut will heal by itself. When you catch a cold, you usually recover in a few days, even without any intervention. Even if you break a bone, the fracture will heal by itself. Soul

Mind Body Medicine works with the body's inherent healing ability, expanding and deepening the potential of your body itself by focusing on the soul as the master healer.

The soul has incredible healing power. But the soul of your body isn't the only soul whose power you can tap in to. Every bodily system has a soul, as does every organ, every cell, and every strand of DNA and RNA.

One of the main treatments in Western medicine is using drugs to adjust the functions of the systems, organs, and cells for healing. Traditional Chinese medicine uses herbs, acupuncture, and *tui na* (Chinese massage) to adjust and heal. Soul Mind Body Medicine adds the power of the soul as a way to adjust and heal the systems, organs, and cells. You only need to know how to connect with the power of your many "inner" souls.

In addition to the inner souls of your body, there are an infinite number of "outer" souls. Animals, oceans, mountains, trees, flowers, buildings, Mother Earth, other planets, the sun, the moon, stars, and galaxies — all have souls. In fact, everything has a soul. All these outer souls have incredible healing power also, and you will learn to use their power to heal soul, mind, and body.

Billions of people believe in the spiritual world. This faith may be expressed through a religion or other belief system. I believe in the Divine (the Creator or the Source) and that, as the creator of the universe, the Divine embraces all religions and belief systems. Buddhas, saints, healing angels, and enlightened masters are all part of the Divine. They all have incredible soul healing power, so they are another incredible healing resource from the universe. We can ask these "outer" souls to heal our soul, mind, and body. Prayer, practiced by many whether or not in the context of a religion, is an application of Soul Power and soul healing. This book will explain the essence of prayer and why it works. It will also give you practical guidance on how to pray most effectively. With the appropriate wisdom and knowledge, you can learn to increase the power of prayer and receive healing miracles from the Divine.

PHYSICAL LIFE AND SPIRITUAL LIFE

The universe can be divided into yin and yang. The yang universe is the physical world we live in. The yin universe is the spiritual world, which comprises all the souls in the universe. Yin and yang are separate, yet connected.

As human beings, we live in the physical world. We conduct our lives and affairs according to the laws of this physical world. Yet whether or not we consciously know or understand it, our souls must follow the laws of the spiritual world. So our physical life is inseparable from our spiritual life, and vice versa. This is becoming increasingly evident as we witness more and more people searching, consciously or subconsciously, for soul wisdom to awaken them and help fulfill their spiritual journeys.

Everyone and everything has a physical life and a spiritual life. A soul or spirit in the universe has a spiritual existence; it has a spiritual life. When a soul returns as a human being, it then has a physical life. Similarly, the sun has both a physical life and a spiritual life. The moon, the planets, and the stars all have their own physical and spiritual lives. Physical life and spiritual life are distinct yet united. They serve each other. Most people are intent on fulfilling their physical lives first. In contrast, Soul Mind Body Medicine teaches you to fulfill your spiritual journey first. You will then receive great benefits for fulfilling your physical life.

> *Heal the soul first; then healing of the mind and body will follow.*
> *Fulfill the soul first; then fulfillment of the mind and body will follow.*

KEY THEORIES

The key theories of Soul Mind Body Medicine are simple, elegant, and easily understood, yet profound in their wisdom and application.

They will give you a clear picture of why people get sick and how they can heal. These theories provide the foundation for the Soul Mind Body Medicine methods for self-healing, healing of others, group healing, and remote healing. Once you learn these methods, you will truly understand the message of Soul Mind Body Medicine:

I have the power to heal myself.
You have the power to heal yourself.
Together we have the power to heal the world.

Once you use the methods of Soul Mind Body Medicine, you will live this message. Let us now explore its underlying theories.

Cell Theory

A body consists of many systems, such as the nervous system, the circulatory system, the digestive system, and the immune system. Each system in turn consists of many organs. For example, the digestive system includes the mouth, esophagus, stomach, small intestine, large intestine, liver, and pancreas. Each organ in turn consists of many cells. Scientists estimate that a brain consists of about 15 billion cells. Each cell is made up of various units such as a nucleus, mitochondria, Golgi apparati, and other organelles. The nucleus includes DNA and RNA. Each cell unit has its specific functions and role. The key points of Cell Theory are as follows:

- A cell is the smallest functioning unit of the body.

- Cells constantly vibrate, expanding and contracting.

- This vibration creates an energy field around each cell.

- Western medicine identifies many causes of illness, including bacteria, viruses, stress, trauma, pollution, and genetic factors. All these factors affect cellular vibration.

- Traditional Chinese medicine identifies many causes of illness, including natural factors such as wind, cold, summer heat, dampness, dryness, and fire; emotional factors such as anger, overexcitement, worry, sadness, and fear; and accidental factors such as falls, snakebites, and injuries. All these factors affect cellular vibration.

- Any cause of illness identified by any healing modality affects cellular vibration. When cellular vibration is affected by any factor posited as a cause of illness, two things can happen: 1) The cells become overactive, radiating lots of energy and increasing the density of the energy around the cells. This energy cannot flow quickly enough through the meridians — the energy pathways, according to traditional Chinese medicine — to other parts of the body, resulting in an energy blockage. 2) The cells become underactive, radiating little energy. This results in an insufficiency of energy around the cells.

- An overaccumulation of energy or, simply, "too much energy" is the root cause of about 85 to 90 percent of all unhealthy conditions. The sicknesses due to "too much energy" include pain, inflammations, cysts, tumors, cancer, and AIDS, as well as emotional imbalances such as anger, depression, anxiety, worry, grief, and fear.

- "Not enough energy" is the root cause of about 10 to 15 percent of sicknesses, including chronic fatigue syndrome and degenerative diseases such as osteoporosis, Alzheimer's, and Parkinson's disease.

- For sicknesses due to "too much energy," the healing solution is to reduce the energy density around the cells. *Soul Mind Body Medicine* will give you practical tools to dissipate and move excess energy around the cells.

- For sicknesses due to "not enough energy," the healing solution is to increase the energy density around the cells. *Soul Mind Body Medicine* will also give you practical tools to increase insufficient energy around the cells.

In one page, the Cell Theory of Soul Mind Body Medicine explains the causes of illness and the nature of healing. Essentially, the rest of this book will give you specific tools and techniques to accomplish healing, both for yourself and others. I will also take you much deeper, into the spiritual aspects of illness and healing, into the *soul* of Soul Mind Body Medicine.

Field Theory

As explained above, a cell constantly vibrates. The energy radiating from the cell's vibration forms a field around the cell. Every cell has its own energy field. Similarly, every organ has its own energy field. The body as a whole has its own energy field, which many people understand as the aura of the body.

According to Soul Mind Body Medicine, the energy fields of all the organs in the body radiate to and influence one another. Illness can also result from imbalances in the energy fields around organs. Just as cells can be over- or underactive, so too can organs. The ultimate healing solution for all illness is to balance the energy fields around every organ and every cell, and to bring all fields into relative balance with each other. To summarize:

- For sicknesses due to "too much energy," the healing solution is to dissipate the density of the fields and reduce the pressure around the organs and cells.

- For sicknesses due to "not enough energy," the healing solution is to increase the density and increase the pressure of the fields around the organs and cells.

Space Theory

There are two kinds of space in the human body. One is the *smaller space*, the space between the cells. The other is the *bigger space*, the space between the organs. Eighty-five to 90 percent of sicknesses are due to having too much energy in the space. Ten to 15 percent of sicknesses are due to not having enough energy in the space.

Energy radiates out from cellular vibration. The collision of these energies happens in the space, both the smaller and the bigger space. Some energies will join together to increase the original energy. Some will join to create new kinds of energy. All these kinds of energy must flow inside the smaller and bigger space. This is very important. Remember that cleaning the energy in the space and promoting energy flow in the space are vital to healing. This book will give you practical tools to reduce or increase the energy density in the space to balance and heal.

Matter Energy Message Theory

A cell consists of a membrane, cytoplasm, and a nucleus. It contains liquid, proteins, cell units, DNA, and RNA. Everything inside the cell is matter.

When a constantly vibrating cell contracts, matter inside the cell transforms to energy outside the cell, in the space around the cell. When a cell expands, energy outside the cell transforms to matter inside the cell. Under normal conditions, this transformation between matter inside the cell and energy outside the cell is in relative balance. If this balance is lost, however, sickness can occur. In fact, any sickness can be explained as an imbalance in the transformation between matter inside the cell and energy outside the cell. The healing solution is to balance this transformation. Soul Mind Body Medicine gives you practical tools to do this, many of which are based on the Matter Energy Message Theory, which states:

> *Message is soul or spirit.*
> *Matter and energy are carriers of message.*
> *Message can directly affect the transformation between*
>   *matter inside the cell and energy outside the cell.*

Message can affect the transformation between matter and energy because it connects with, directs, and balances both matter and energy. A prayer is a message. Therefore, prayer can affect the transformation between matter and energy, which means that prayer can heal.

This wisdom clearly explains how and why prayer works. It really is that simple. A great deal of scientific research, not to mention anecdotal evidence, has demonstrated that prayer works, but scientists haven't been able to explain clearly how. Matter Energy Message Theory explains how prayer works because it makes it clear that message works at the cellular level and at the DNA and RNA level, directly affecting both the matter inside the cells and the energy outside the cells. Message can balance the transformation between matter inside the cells and energy outside the cells.

This wisdom reveals the essence of how spiritual healing can work for the physical body, emotional body, and mental body. The Matter Energy Message Theory can explain any cause of illness from the perspective of all kinds of medicine. It is a universal law, representing the essence of soul healing. The most powerful methods of Soul Mind Body Medicine are applications of this theory.

Most other healing modalities focus on matter, as Western medicine does, or on energy. Many healing modalities take it one step further, by connecting the mind and the body. Even Western medicine now acknowledges, studies, and uses the power of the mind-body connection in healing. However, very rarely does any healing modality pay sufficient attention to the soul.

The soul's power is profound. Very rarely does healing really explain and use the *soul-energy-matter* connection, which is another way to express the *matter-energy-message* connection. Only fairly recently in this modern world, with its high stress and its materialistic culture, have soul issues begun to earn greater attention. But people still do not have much soul wisdom, despite their growing desire, even yearning, for it. In this book I offer some of the deepest and simplest techniques of Soul Power, not only for healing, but for every aspect of your life. The simplest secrets are the best secrets. Keep that wisdom in mind as I share them with you throughout this book.

Some Tips for Reading

Before moving on to the remaining key theories of Soul Mind Body Medicine, let me share some of simplest and best secrets that you can apply as you read this book. In fact, these are simple but profound tips for reading *any* book. When you read, sit down straight. Put the tip of your tongue close to, but not touching, the roof of your mouth. Contract your anus a little, and tuck in your lower abdomen. Maintain this position while you read. Why? This is the greatest meditation for boosting energy, healing, and rejuvenation.

Every gem of wisdom and knowledge, every practice, every sentence of this book is a message. These messages have immeasurable healing and blessing power to balance the matter inside cells and the energy outside cells. When you maintain this reading position, your cells will be in a state of inner peace, awareness, and relaxation. Whatever part of this book you are reading, your cells will be open to receive the healing and blessings simultaneously. Read slowly. Comprehend and digest and absorb well. From now on, use this reading technique. Every word has a soul. Every sentence has a soul. A soul carries love, light, healing, blessing, and service. This reading secret can dramatically transform every aspect of your life.

Conservation of Energy

Another key theory of Soul Mind Body Medicine is the Law of the Conservation of Energy. This law of physics states that energy can never be lost; it can only transform from one form to another. Energy can transform to matter, and matter can transform to energy, but energy can never disappear.

Consider the clouds in the sky. The water from the oceans (*di chi*, or Earth energy) transforms to water vapor, which is one kind of energy. As the water vapor rises, it becomes clouds (*tian chi*, or Heaven energy). Then, the energy from the heavens descends in the form of rain, another kind of energy. Although these are all different forms of energy, the energy is always conserved.

A stone erodes naturally due to wind and rain. The stone becomes smaller and smaller. If a stone is struck at the same point for hundreds of years by dripping water, a hole will form in the stone and, eventually, through the stone. The part of the stone that has eroded away to leave a hole is the part that has turned to another form of energy in the universe. Similarly, when a human being dies and is buried, the energy is absorbed by Mother Earth and then transforms into other forms of energy. *Soul Mind Body Medicine* will give you practical techniques for transforming energy to heal.

THE CAUSES OF ILLNESS

Now let's move to the key theories of Soul Mind Body Medicine regarding illness. In Western medicine, some of the causes of illness include bacteria, viruses, parasites, stress, trauma, physical defects in organs such as the heart, biochemical imbalances in the brain, environmental factors, and genetic factors. There are many others. According to traditional Chinese medicine, illnesses are caused by an imbalance of yin and yang or of the Five Elements — Wood, Fire, Earth, Metal, and Water. The body's systems, organs, and tissues can be categorized by these elements, which are interrelated and interdependent. Put simply, if they are balanced, one is healthy. When the balance is lost, one is sick. As we know, Soul Mind Body Medicine groups the causes of illness into three types:

- energy blockage
- matter blockage
- spiritual blockage

All illnesses, whether of the physical, emotional, mental, or spiritual body, are caused by one or more of these blockages. This very simple characterization of the causes of illness is a key reason why Soul Mind Body Medicine can offer practical tools for healing any condition. Let's explore each of these blockages in turn.

Energy Blockages

Why do people get sick? Five thousand years ago, the *Yellow Emperor's Canon*, the ancient authoritative text of traditional Chinese medicine, stated: "If chi flows, one is healthy. If chi is blocked, one is sick."

What *is* chi? The word *chi* means "vital energy" or "life force," as in tai chi and qi gong. In traditional Chinese medicine, there are at least fifty chis, for example, heart chi, liver chi, kidney chi, ying chi, wei chi. Most people have no concept of all these types of chi. It takes five years of hard, serious study to learn traditional Chinese medicine. It would take you a long time just to learn all the different chis in traditional Chinese medicine. I honor this wisdom. But for the purposes of this book my teaching is: *There is only one chi in the universe.*

The energy radiating out from the heart is called heart chi. The energy radiating out from the immune system is called the chi of the immune system. The energy radiating out from the cells is called cell chi. The energy radiating out from the body and the blood vessels is called wei chi. The energy radiating out from a tree is named tree chi. The energy radiating out from the ocean is named ocean chi. The energy radiating out from the stars is named star chi. In one sentence, the energy radiating out from anyone or anything is named the chi of that person or that thing.

But everyone and everything is in the universe. Everyone and everything radiates the chi of the universe. That's why every kind of chi is universal chi. We can take this even further. There are countless universes. There are countless chi's of countless universes. Universes can be divided as yang universes, which are the physical worlds, and yin universes, which are the spiritual worlds. The Divine creates the yang and yin universes. Yang and yin universes radiate divine chi. The Divine is one. All universes are one. That is why I state that there is only one chi.

Let's return to our question: Why do people get sick? According to Soul Mind Body Medicine, the root cause of most illness is energy blockages. This concept synthesizes some ideas of Western medicine and traditional Chinese medicine. Western medicine talks about the cell, while traditional Chinese medicine talks about chi. Soul Mind Body Medicine puts the two together, by saying that *illness is caused by chi blockage at the cellular level.*

How does chi get blocked? As I explained, cells consist of matter. When cells contract, matter inside the cells turns into energy outside of the cells. When cells expand, the energy outside the cells transforms into matter inside the cells. Health depends on a relative balance in this transformation between matter and energy at the cellular level. It doesn't matter what Western medicine or traditional Chinese medicine — or any healing modality — identifies as the causes of illness. In the end, the effect is always seen at the cellular level, in the form of an imbalance in the transformation between matter and energy. If that transformation is not balanced, then sickness occurs, no matter what other cause has been identified. If that transformation can remain in relative balance, sickness will not occur, even in the presence of other "causes" of illness. This balance will naturally prevent sickness and maintain optimum health.

Matter-Energy Transformation

Let me explain the matter-energy transformation in more detail.

As we know, cells contract and expand constantly. There are many processes like this in your body. Think about your lungs. The act of breathing, of inhaling and exhaling, alternates between expansion and contraction. Think about digestion. After you eat, your stomach cells contract and expand. Then the food goes to your small intestine, whose cells also contract and expand. At this very moment, as you are focused on reading this book, your brain cells are contracting and expanding. Contraction and expansion is a law of cellular vibration.

How do we understand that there is only one chi? Because chi is simply the energy radiating out from the vibration of matter. When cells vibrate, they are contracting and expanding, radiating chi. When cells contract, matter inside the cells transforms into energy that radiates out to the space between the cells and outside the cells. After contracting, cells will then expand. When cells expand, the energy between the cells will transform back into matter inside the cells. When you are healthy, the transformation between matter and energy at the cellular level is in relative balance.

In Western medicine, a virus causes you to catch the flu. It enters

12

your lungs, you come down with a fever and have a cough, headaches, and sore muscles, and you may take a week or so to recover. Some people may develop further problems, such as bronchitis or pneumonia. Some may even develop a kidney infection as a reaction. But in traditional Chinese medicine, it is energy — always energy — that makes you sick. In the view of Soul Mind Body Medicine, what has happened? Initially, the virus simply affected the vibration of the cells in the bronchial tubes and the lungs. The virus stimulated these cells, causing them to be too active, to overcontract, causing lots of energy to radiate out. This high density or accumulation of energy remains between the cells, because the energy cannot flow quickly enough to other parts of the body, nor can it transform into matter quickly enough. The energy is literally stuck. It is blocked between the cells. This leads to coughing, inflammation, pain, and other problems.

Some people may have chronic inflammation caused by anger and other emotional imbalances. Some people may be chronically uncomfortable or constantly tired and stressed. Later, they may have pain or discomfort in their stomach. They go to the doctor, get examined, but nothing shows up. Six months later, perhaps, the pain and discomfort persist, but still no physical changes can be seen or measured. Then, when they go to the doctor to get checked again, maybe one year later, they find something growing inside the stomach. That is an example of why a tumor or cancer takes time to develop. Anger, stress, and many other emotions and issues can make your cells overactive. Matter inside the cells turns into lots of energy around the cells. This "excess" energy cannot flow fast enough to other parts of the body, nor can it completely transform back into matter. The transformation between matter inside the cells and energy outside the cells is quite unbalanced.

Matter Blockages

Many illnesses can also be considered the result of a matter blockage. Of course, matter blockages and energy blockages are closely related, through the matter-energy transformation at the cellular level.

When any factor makes cellular vibration overactive anywhere in the body, the energy radiating out from these cells accumulates because it cannot flow quickly enough to other parts of the body. Meanwhile, through the capillary system, the cells are constantly receiving nutrients, or more matter. This matter cannot transform to energy outside the cells because of the high pressure of the accumulated energy outside the cells. This results in *too much matter* in the cells.

The opposite imbalance occurs when there is *not enough matter* in the cells. Some people have a poor appetite, or problems digesting and absorbing food and nutrients well. This lack of matter and deficiency of nutrients leads to biochemical changes affecting all the body's systems. Anemia, for example, is a literal lack of matter in the form of red blood cells. Often, people who are very weak, such as after major surgery, who have lost a lot of blood, or who have suffered chronically from indigestion and poor absorption will not have enough matter inside the cells.

Spiritual Blockages

Spiritual blockages are the result of mistakes you have made in previous lives and in your current life. These mistakes are recorded in the spiritual world as bad karma, also known as bad *te* (pronounced "duh"), which means "bad virtue" or "bad deeds." Any harmful acts, behaviors, and even thoughts that you create, including killing, harming, stealing, and cheating, will add to your bad karma. All the activities, behaviors, and thoughts of one's life are recorded in the Akashic Records, or the Book of Life, which contains the history of every soul in the universe since creation.

Karma, which means the "record of services," can be divided into good and bad. Service that benefits humanity and the universe is categorized as good karma. Service that harms humanity and the universe is categorized as bad karma. Spiritual law clearly states: a person with good karma will receive blessings from the spiritual world, including good health, relationships, finances, family, and every aspect of life. A person with bad karma will pay a price and learn lessons. Bad karma is the root of blockages and disasters in every aspect of life.

You may or may not believe in karma. I fully respect whatever you believe. I have no intention of making you a believer. What I am doing here is sharing my personal knowledge and spiritual wisdom. As human beings in the physical world, we are subject to the laws of our country, state, and city. When we break these laws, we may become involved with lawyers and judges. You may not realize that your soul, my soul, every soul is subject to the spiritual laws of the universe. And, just as there are lawyers and judges in the physical world, there are lawyers and judges in the spiritual world.

When does karma affect one's life? The effects of karma could appear instantly, or in years, or even lifetimes. If you are very disciplined and committed to serving humanity, your bad karma will be cleansed. Its effects will be softened and postponed. Potential disasters in your life can be deferred or even averted. The spiritual world will give you more time to completely clear your karma. The more you serve, the more blessings you will receive. When you offer good service, you are extremely blessed in every aspect of your life.

On the other hand, if you do not realize that bad karma needs to be cleansed and you continually do unpleasant things, then blockages and disasters will come to every aspect of your life, including health, relationships, finances, and family. Think about yourself. Evaluate every aspect of your life. Some parts of your life are clearly blessed. Some parts of your life may not be. Correct your mistakes. Offer pure service to transform your life. (By evaluating your life, you can figure out how much good service you have offered in previous lives. In turn, the good service you offer in your current life will directly influence your future lives.)

It should be obvious that I believe deeply in reincarnation, from my personal experience and my open spiritual channels. You may not believe in it, and that is fine. I'm not here to impose my belief system on anyone. I honor everyone's beliefs. But I am convinced that when we die, our soul goes to the universe, and later it will return. Up down, up down — every soul goes up and comes back down to begin another life.

The law of karma is epitomized by this famous statement from ancient Chinese spiritual teaching: *Heaven is the most fair*. For example, parents who honor, respect, and love their own parents a great deal will generally have children who love and honor them. On the other hand, people who do not treat their parents properly or lovingly will generally receive similar treatment from their own children. Karma is the reason why the Golden Rule can be found in a wide range of cultures and spiritual traditions across the planet, and why it is absolutely correct. *Do unto others as you would have them do unto you*, because if you give love to others, generally speaking, you will receive love in return. If you argue with, disrespect, abuse, or hate others, you will receive conflict, disharmony, and bad treatment in return.

Spiritual blockages or bad karma are the root blockages in life. Serious, chronic, and life-threatening illnesses typically are karma related. Inability to achieve a successful romantic relationship, automobile accidents, and constant business failures could all be karma related. Think about your own life and the lives of your loved ones and friends. Do any of them make the same mistakes or encounter the same blockages again and again in their personal lives, their careers, or their family and romantic relationships? Why do they have the same illness over and over? Why do they suffer from chronic health problems for years? Why are they "stuck" in the same patterns? Why do some of them have such "bad luck"? The answer is karma. This is the lesson to be learned by each person.

If you are on a spiritual journey, you are searching for deep soul wisdom. This wisdom about karma is a key in making any spiritual journey. When you learn how to cleanse bad karma and remove spiritual blockages with Soul Mind Body Medicine, your life will be absolutely transformed.

DIAGNOSING ILLNESS

Western medicine uses many diagnostic approaches, including various physical examinations, such as palpitation, blood and urine tests,

X-rays, CT scans, and MRIs. Traditional Chinese medicine has its own diagnostic approaches, including pulse reading, tongue reading, stool reading, smelling the patient, and other methods. I honor the theories, diagnostic approaches, and healing methods of all medicines and healing modalities. However, Soul Mind Body Medicine offers its own unique diagnostic approaches, which we'll explore below.

Diagnosing Energy Imbalances

As I have explained, there are only two kinds of energy imbalances that can result in sickness. One is *too much energy* between the cells, in the space. The other is *not enough energy* between the cells, in the space. Diagnosis is simple: *any* kind of pain or inflammation, all cysts and tumors, cancer, AIDS, and most emotional imbalances, including anger, depression, anxiety, worry, grief, and fear, are due to too much energy around the cells or around the organs.

How many kinds of pain are there? How many kinds of inflammation? How many kinds of tumors and cancers? In the view of Soul Mind Body Medicine, if you suffer from any of these conditions, it doesn't matter where your pain is located. It doesn't matter what the nature of the pain is. It doesn't matter what kind of cancer you have, or what stage it is in. All these conditions are caused by excess or *too much energy* in the space. About 85 to 90 percent of all sicknesses on the physical, emotional, mental, and spiritual levels fall into this category.

Any kind of degenerative change and chronic fatigue are due to *not enough energy* around the cells or around the organs. For example, degenerative changes in the muscles or tissues, in the bones (osteoporosis), in the brain (Alzheimer's), Parkinson's disease, multiple sclerosis, chronic fatigue syndrome, and fibromyalgia are all caused by insufficient or *not enough energy* in the space. About 10 to 15 percent of all sicknesses on the physical, emotional, mental, and spiritual levels fall into this category.

The great simplicity of diagnosis in Soul Mind Body Medicine results in great simplicity in healing. The healing solution for illnesses caused by *too much energy* is to dissipate the excess energy. The healing solution for illnesses caused by *not enough energy* is to increase or build up the energy. *Soul Mind Body Medicine* will give you simple and practical tools to support both solutions.

Diagnosing Matter Imbalances

As we've discussed, matter imbalances are closely related to energy imbalances, owing to the matter-energy transformation at the cellular level. Because of this relationship, when using Soul Mind Body Medicine you may not need to diagnose the matter imbalance, so long as you can diagnose an energy imbalance. However, like almost everything in Soul Mind Body Medicine, it is not at all difficult to tell whether a person suffers from *too much matter* or *not enough matter*, thanks to this tool: checking the tongue. The character of the tongue reveals the condition of matter in the body. If you have a thick, big tongue, you have *too much matter* inside the cells. If your tongue is very thin, tiny, or pale, you have *not enough matter* inside the cells.

Diagnosing Spiritual Blockages

Generally speaking, Western healthcare professionals do not consider, much less identify, spiritual blockages. To be able to identify them, a healer must do Xiu Lian to open his or her spiritual channels. When the spiritual channels are open, one can then determine a person's spiritual blockages.

Xiu Lian (pronounced "shew lien") is an ancient term for the spiritual journey, for the purification of soul, mind, and body through meditation, chanting, and other practices. Xiu Lian includes training the body (to promote the internal flow of energy and blood, as well as external flexibility), training the consciousness (to purify thought and gain Mind Power), training the heart (to open it fully to love, compassion, kindness, and pure service to humanity), and training the soul (to purify the soul, develop your soul's warehouse of intelligence, and uplift your spiritual standing). The wisdom, knowledge, and practices of Xiu Lian are vast. The healing meditations in chapter 5 and, in fact, all the healing exercises in this book can be considered Xiu Lian.

Xiu Lian will develop your spiritual channels, enabling you to identify spiritual blockages. If you cannot do this yet, that's perfectly okay. You can use and benefit fully from Soul Mind Body Medicine without this ability.

EVERYONE IS A HEALER

Soul Mind Body Medicine empowers you to heal yourself and others. The basis for this is not complicated. Everyone is a natural healer. If you cut yourself, the wound heals by itself. If you catch a cold, you will recover in a few days. All the systems of the body — the immune system, the cardiovascular system, the nervous system, and so on — have self-regenerating and self-healing abilities. All the organs and all the cells have the same abilities. If they coordinate these abilities well, they can heal your physical, emotional, mental, and spiritual conditions.

In order to heal one has to relax. This is the most important requirement for healing. When you are tense and tight, your cells, in turn, will be tense and tight. Cellular vibration will be abnormal, and this will affect the functions, coordination, and balance of the organs and systems. This imbalance sustains illness and impedes healing. I cannot emphasize strongly enough: relaxation is the most important requirement in healing. Only when you are relaxed can your cells vibrate actively and in balance. When this happens, healing is supported and promoted.

Second, everyone is a healer because we all can use the mind to heal. Positive thinking, creative visualization, imagery, meditation, intention, concentration, and manifestation — all these capabilities of the mind fall under Mind Power. In chapter 3, "Mind Over Matter," I will share some powerful approaches that will give you great Mind Power for healing.

Third, the most important and powerful healing technique available to everyone is using the soul. The soul has incredible power for healing, but how many people know how to use and develop Soul

Power? In chapter 2, "Soul Over Matter," you will learn one of the simplest, yet one of the most powerful, approaches of soul healing: Say Hello Healing. Using the power of the soul to heal is the heart — and soul — of Soul Mind Body Medicine.

Everyone *is* a healer. But once you learn how to use the power of the mind and the power of the soul to heal, together with the many specific healing techniques I will introduce in this book, your healing ability will increase dramatically.

Healing Power

Soul Mind Body Medicine is energy and spiritual healing, or soul healing. It does not require that you master a vast body of knowledge or that you spend years in internships and clinical practice.

Your natural healing power is your *soul* healing power. What determines your Soul Power? It depends on your spiritual standing. In my understanding, there are nine layers of Heaven, which is why I refer to Heaven as the Jiu Tian (literally, the "nine heavens"). Your soul stands on one of these nine levels, as does every human being's soul. The higher your soul's standing, the greater your healing power. Why? When you offer a healing to others or even to yourself, the higher your spiritual standing, the more assistance you will receive from the spiritual world. The higher your spiritual standing, the higher and more powerful the saints, healing angels, Buddhas, ascended masters, and spiritual masters and leaders in Heaven who will assist your healing.

How do we increase our spiritual standing? The key is purification. Purify your soul, mind, and body. Service is vital. Serve humanity unconditionally. When you serve humanity, Mother Earth, or the universe, your service is recorded in the Akashic Records as good virtue or karma. When you have accumulated a sufficient amount of virtue, your spiritual standing will be uplifted, and your healing power will increase.

Healing power can be given to you by a physical enlightened master or by the spiritual saints, Buddhas, healing angels, or other high beings in the soul world. In other words, healing power can be given to you by a divine channel or directly from the Divine.

Whether in physical or spiritual form, an enlightened master can transmit healing power to students who are ready, who are totally committed to serving humanity unconditionally. Generally speaking, such a master will give serious tests to devoted students. These tests could be challenges in any aspect of life, including health, relationships, business, and emotions. When the master confirms that the student has passed the tests, he or she will transmit healing power to the student. Real healing power comes from Soul Power.

We are ready now to examine Soul Power in greater depth.

Soul Over Matter

This chapter is the essence of Soul Mind Body Medicine. In it I will reveal some of the deepest wisdom of the soul. You will learn such basics as what the soul is and what its characteristics are. You will understand how the soul, mind, and body are related. And you will grasp the essence of soul healing: how the soul can heal your soul, mind, and body and how the soul of nature can heal you. You will learn the Law of Universal Service, which is a golden key to healing. After you have built this foundation, the rest of this book will give you the practical tools of Soul Mind Body Medicine for applying this deepest wisdom to heal yourself, others, society, and the universe.

BASIC SOUL WISDOM

We know about the wisdom of the mind, about its potential to transform our life. We now understand how the mind can be used for healing and blessing, through guided imagery, creative visualization, meditation, positive thinking, confidence, creativity, and flexibility. Scientific research has turned up more and more evidence of the mind's capacity to work wonders in health and healing. Over the course of a few decades, the mind-body connection has evolved from heresy to conventional wisdom. *Mind over matter* has become a cliché.

These days, we constantly hear about the body, mind, and soul or spirit. So why do I list the soul, mind, and body in that order? With Soul Mind Body Medicine I am introducing the power of the soul, or *soul over matter*. Yes, the mind is powerful, but the soul is *much more* powerful. The soul can work wonders that the mind can barely grasp.

What Is the Soul?

I once saw a newspaper article with the headline "Does a company have a soul?" I could only chuckle. Of course a company has a soul! *Everything* has a soul. A human being has a soul. An animal has a soul. A flower or a tree has a soul. Living things have a soul. Inanimate things have a soul. A stone has a soul. Everything in the universe has a soul.

Soul is the same as spirit. In China and India, people talk a lot about the soul. In the West, people talk more about the spirit. Western science studies the messages of the cells and the communication between cells and organs. In fact, "soul," "spirit," and "message" are just different names for the same thing. The soul is the essence of life. For anything in the universe, the soul is the essence of that thing.

Where is the soul located? For human beings, it is located in the lower abdomen. After you open your spiritual channels, especially your Third Eye, you will be able to see your soul in your lower abdomen, confirming that it is a real entity inside your body. (The Third Eye, one of the body's major spiritual centers, is a cherry-sized energy center located in the center of your head. When you develop and open the Third Eye, you will be able to see images of the spiritual world. In chapter 8, I will give you an exercise to develop and open the Third Eye.)

Further, your soul can move around within your body. With advanced training, your soul can even emerge from its physical tent and travel through the universe. Similarly, the soul of an inanimate thing is located within that thing. A person's soul resembles the person. An animal's soul looks like the animal. The soul of an inanimate object also looks like that object. Again, for those people who have developed their spiritual capabilities, all these souls are visible. Of course, for most people, souls remain invisible.

This is not new wisdom. Thousands of years ago, ancient Chinese spiritual teaching held that everything, including inanimate things, has a soul. But what Soul Mind Body Medicine does is *use* the power of all these souls for healing. Once you learn the tools of soul healing, you will be able to apply them easily and effectively.

Soul Concepts

Without going too deeply into details here, I want to enumerate some of the characteristics of the soul to give you an idea of the limitlessness of soul wisdom. I will focus more on this topic in my forthcoming *Soul Wisdom* book series.[1] And later in this book I will elaborate on some of the deepest soul secrets for healing, which are at the core of Soul Mind Body Medicine.

- *The soul is an independent entity inside your body*. For most people, the soul is located in the Lower Dan Tian, a fist-sized energy center in your lower abdomen.[2] After you open your Third Eye, you can see your own soul, which will look like a little figure sitting there.

- *The soul has its own will, thoughts, and preferences*. Your soul may want to do certain things very strongly. It may have very clear likes and dislikes.

- *The soul has emotions and feelings*. Your soul can be happy, depressed, excited, calm, or irritated. Just as your brain holds memories, so too does your soul. Your soul can remember many things from its past lives.

- *The soul has creativity*. Your mind can create, but your soul can create even more.

- *The soul has flexibility*. Your soul can help you overcome many difficulties. Love your soul. Ask it to bless your life. This is an example of *soul over matter*.

- *The soul can communicate*. Your soul communicates with other souls on its own. You can communicate with your own soul. In fact, you are in constant communication with your soul, albeit not consciously. Your mind could say, "My dear soul, I want to do something. Would you like that too?" Your soul could respond, "Yes, I would like that."

- *The soul possesses incredible wisdom*. Your soul's wisdom comes from experiences and memories of its hundreds, perhaps thousands, of lives. Just as your mind is constantly learning, so too is your soul. Your soul loves to learn and is searching for new knowledge all the time. Your soul may travel when you are asleep to learn from your spiritual guides and teachers. The key to tapping into this great wisdom is to be able to communicate with your soul *consciously*. When your spiritual channels are open, you can converse with your soul. You will be amazed at how much your soul knows. It has great wisdom and could become your best consultant.

- *The soul can heal*. Your soul can heal your mind and body. It can prevent sickness. It can protect your life. How do we apply Soul Power to heal? It is very simple: say *hello* to your soul. Honor your soul. Appreciate your soul. Ask it to bless your healing. This book will teach you exactly how to do this.

THE RELATIONSHIP OF
SOUL, MIND, AND BODY

To review, a human being consists of soul, mind, and body. Soul is spirit or message, which is the essence of life. The mind can be separated between the subconscious mind, which is the deep mind, and the conscious mind, which is the superficial mind. The body consists of all the systems, organs, and cells.

Your soul, mind, and body are in constant communication with each other. Your soul gives an order and direction to your subconscious mind; the subconscious mind passes the order and direction to your conscious mind. The final decision is made by your conscious mind, but it has been directed to the conscious mind by your soul.

Your subconscious mind may not agree with the soul. In this case, your subconscious mind says, "No, I don't want to do that," sending this message to your conscious mind. If your conscious mind says, "Great, I agree with you. I don't want to do it either," then you and your mind are not in harmony with your soul. Your subconscious mind and your conscious mind do not follow the direction of your soul.

You may think, "I have the freedom to do whatever I want." Yes, I agree. You have free will. But I want to share a deep spiritual truth: when you decide to do something, your conscious mind connects with your subconscious mind and your soul. Your mind may want to do something, but it doesn't mean your soul wants to do the same thing. When you plan to do something that your soul agrees with, things will go much more smoothly than they would if your soul disagreed. If your conscious mind, your subconscious mind, and your soul are all in agreement, then your decision will be blessed — smooth, peaceful, happy, and successful — whether it involves your business, your relationships, your spiritual journey, or your healing journey. If you make a decision that your soul disagrees with, many problems — I call them "blockages" — will occur. Things will not be smooth, peaceful, or successful. Your soul creates these problems for you because it is not happy. *The soul is the boss!*

FOOD FOR THE SOUL

Human beings need food to survive, and so do souls. What is food for the soul? The answer is *virtue*. In Taoist practice, virtue is called *te*. In Buddhist practice, it is called karma. In Western religions, people refer to deeds. Karma, *te*, deed, and virtue are different names for the same thing. They are the record of services. This record includes the good — karma, *te*, deed, virtue — and the bad. Good virtue is food and nourishment for your soul. Bad virtue harms your soul and blocks your journey.

Good karma or virtue is created by acts of love, care, compassion, sincerity, honesty, integrity, generosity, purity, charity, volunteerism, prayer, healing, and unconditional service. Bad karma or virtue is created by harmful acts, such as killing, harming, being deceitful, lying, being jealous, being greedy, and being selfish. Behaviors and thoughts, as well as actions, can create karma, both good and bad.

Why should you want good food for your soul? Good karma can absolutely bless your life, giving you happiness, health, peace, and harmony. It can transform your life and help you reach soul enlightenment. Bad karma can lead to suffering, unhappiness, and blockages in many aspects of your life, including your relationships with family members, friends, colleagues, and your environment. It can affect your business, your health, and even your life span.

With good virtue as food, the soul becomes purer, more loving, kinder, gentler, more peaceful, and happier. Think about the people you know who are pure, loving, gentle, and tender. You may also know people who are rude, unpleasant, dishonest, and intolerant. These people have fed their souls the food of bad virtue. These are two different kinds of people, because their souls are different from eating different soul foods.

When you open your Third Eye, you will know whether someone has good virtue just by looking at his or her soul. If the soul is fat, beautiful, relaxed, and happy, that person has very good virtue. If the soul is thin and looks unpleasant, miserable, sad, or angry, that person is lacking in virtue or *te*; he or she has created much bad karma and has therefore had a lot of bad nourishment.

SAY HELLO HEALING

It is time for me to reveal one of the simplest yet one of the most sacred and powerful techniques of Soul Mind Body Medicine. This technique, which can be used for self-healing, healing others, group healing, and remote or distant healing, represents the essence of soul healing. I call it Say Hello Healing.

When you leave your home in the morning to catch a bus or a train for work, or perhaps to go for a walk first, you say "good morning" to your neighbors. On the bus or train, you say "hello" to your fellow commuters. As you leave work at the end of the day, you say "have a good evening" to your colleagues. Stopping in at your local market on the way home, you say "how are you?" to your favorite clerk. Before you go to sleep, you say "good night" to your family. You understand how to "say hello" in daily life. In Soul Mind Body Medicine, saying hello is just as simple. All you need to do is to request your soul to heal your soul, mind, and body.

Say Hello to Inner Souls

As we explored in the last chapter, there are two kinds of souls you can call on for healing — the "inner" and the "outer" souls. Your inner souls are your own (your body's) soul, the souls of your systems, organs, cells, DNA, and RNA. Your own soul and the souls of your systems, organs, and cells have both the power and wisdom to heal themselves and to heal you.

Say Hello Healing is simple and direct. Just say hello, express your love and appreciation, and make your request. For example, if you are suffering from back pain, say: *Dear soul of my back, I love you. Could you offer a healing to my back? You have the power to heal yourself. Do a good job. Thank you.* Then relax your body completely. Remain relaxed for three minutes. See what happens. You may receive a "miracle" healing. You may feel much better. You may feel a little better. You may feel nothing at all. Just because you feel nothing or don't notice any improvement, that doesn't mean Say Hello Healing doesn't work. After all, you've only spent a few minutes trying to relieve some pain that may have been bothering you for hours, even days. This technique may be too simple for you to believe. All I ask is that you keep an open mind and try it a few more times, perhaps for a few more days.

I have taught this technique to many people worldwide, and a large majority of them reported that they have benefited from it. I have also experienced the results personally. I believe that this is the time to share these techniques with all of humanity and with the entire universe. Give Say Hello Healing a try. It may not work right away, but that doesn't mean it won't ever work. You may have been sick for months or even years, especially if you have chronic pain or a life-threatening condition. Be patient. The blockages causing the illness may have been created over an extended period of time. Be sincere. Be confident. Be persistent. Open your heart, your mind, and your soul to receive healing from the universe.

Healing Formula for Soul Power

In saying hello to your inner souls, you can use a simple formula, like the one provided above in the example of healing back pain. Despite its simplicity, this formula carries incredible healing wisdom and deep spiritual secrets. It consists of five sentences:

> Say hello: *Dear soul, mind, and body of my* _____,
> Give love: *I love you.*
> Make an affirmation: *You have the power to heal yourself.*
> Give an order: *Do a good job!*
> Express gratitude and courtesy: *Thank you.*

Remember these five sentences for every healing situation. We will follow this formula throughout the rest of this book.

When you say hello in the first sentence, the order in which you speak to the soul, mind, and body is very important. If you need healing for your heart, for example, be sure to say, "Dear soul, mind, and body of my heart," and not "Dear body, mind, and soul of my heart" or "Dear mind, soul, and body of my heart." Soul comes first because it is the essence of life. It is the boss. Understand and communicate with your soul. Ask it to give you healing and blessings. Then enjoy the results.

Say Hello to Outer Souls

The second group of souls you can call on for healing is your "outer" souls — the souls of nature, the healing angels, the Buddhas, the saints, your ancestors, and your loved ones — or whoever fits in with your beliefs. You can say hello to anything in the universe and ask it to heal you. *Every* soul has the power to give you a healing. Here is how to ask for it:

Dear soul of the sun, I love you. Could you offer a healing to my painful shoulder? Thank you.

Dear soul of Mother Earth, I love you. Could you heal my feet? Thank you.

Dear souls of the stars, I love you. Could you give me kidney power? Thank you.

Dear souls of the healing angels, I love you. Could you give me a blessing to boost my immunity? Thank you.

We, as human beings, have physical form. Many great, enlightened beings serve us while they are in soul form. You may recognize many of them, such as Jesus, Mary, Guan Yin (the Goddess of Compassion), Lao Tzu, and others. There are many, many more saints, Buddhas, and ascended masters you may not be familiar with. After you open your Third Eye, you will be able to see them. You will see that, like us, they wear clothes, they smile. Though formless, these enlightened teachers serve you. They have been in the spiritual world for thousands of years. When you call on any of these outer souls, they will serve and bless you. If you need them, pray to them, and they will be there for you.

Say Hello Healing recognizes that unlimited healing powers and capabilities are available twenty-four hours a day, seven days a week. All you need to do is to say hello to them. Be very honored and calm. Totally relax to receive the blessing. If you are sensitive, you will actually feel the healing light, love, and energy, in the form of tingling, waves, heat, or coolness. Some people with open spiritual channels will see spiritual healing light, or soul light, or even the saints and Buddhas themselves. Regardless of what you can feel or see, you will be amazed that healing can be so simple.

Gratitude Is Key

Say Hello Healing is one of the simplest and most powerful healing techniques that I am sharing with you in this book. I do not expect to convince everyone. But because you, dear reader, have come this far with me, I hope you will be willing to open your mind and give it a try. If it works, you are blessed. Be most grateful to the souls who have responded to your request. If it doesn't work right away, as I have said, be patient and confident. Don't give up! Try to be grateful, whatever result you receive. If Say Hello Healing just does not work for you, then please forget it.

Remember, after you say hello and make your healing request, calm down completely for three to five minutes, to receive the healing blessing from the soul you addressed. If you want to practice longer, that's great — the longer, the better. When you completely relax, your cells, organs, and systems will be more open to receive the healing blessing. The transformation between matter inside the cells and energy outside the cells will be balanced, and the energy or matter blockages causing your unhealthy condition will be removed. You will be restored to health.

When you are done receiving the healing blessing, remember to say, "Thank you. Thank you. Thank you." The first "thank you" is for the Divine. The second "thank you" is for the soul or souls you requested help from. The third "thank you" is for your own soul. Thank the Divine because everything comes from the Divine. Everything is part of the Divine. Thank the souls you requested help from because they gave you their love, light, and healing blessing. Thank your own inner souls because you were open-minded enough to receive the blessing that you requested. (If you are not truly open to receiving the healing, you will receive a lesser blessing.) Gratitude is a key spiritual courtesy, no less important and beneficial than showing gratitude and courtesy to others in our everyday lives. It is appreciated and recognized by the soul world no less than it is by your fellow human beings.

I give my love, my heart, and my service to you unconditionally by sharing this healing wisdom with you. I hope you will practice Say Hello Healing every day. There is no time limit on its use. You can practice anywhere, anytime. Whenever you need it, whenever you ask for it, the energy of the universe will bless you. Dear Divine, the entire universe, everyone, please bless this special servant, Say Hello Healing. Thank you. Thank you. Thank you.

UNIVERSAL SERVICE

How can you make Say Hello Healing — or any healing — more powerful and effective? The deepest healing and blessing wisdom is to offer universal service unconditionally. Everything and everyone — a dog, a cat, a tree, an ocean, a mountain, a house, the sun, and the moon — is a universal servant. Everything and everyone serves the universe in its own way, offering universal love, forgiveness, peace, healing, blessing, harmony, and enlightenment.

Offer as much unconditional service as you can to benefit others, animals, nature, society, and the universe. Try your best to serve more. The more service you can give to the universe, the more blessings you will receive in return. You may not receive material rewards, but you will gain lots of virtue. This virtue or good karma will absolutely bless your spiritual life and your healing journey.

When acting as a universal servant, remember that love and forgiveness are the keys to healing. Love melts all blockages. Forgiveness brings peace and inner joy. Let's explore these keys below.

LOVE MELTS ANY BLOCKAGE

Every religion, every spiritual teacher, teaches love. It is the key to spiritual study. It is the key to life. It is the key to the universe.

The example of unconditional love that everyone can relate to is a mother's love for her children. What about unconditional love in religious teaching? In Buddhist teaching, for example, there are many Buddhas. They are all universal servants. Many people know and revere Guan Shi Yin Buddha (Guan Yin), the Goddess of Compassion. Guan means "observe." Shi means "world." Yin means "action and voice." So literally, Guan Shi Yin means "observe the world's actions and hear the world's voice."

Guan Yin, who gives unconditional love to the universe, is honored by many millions of followers. Countless people throughout history have called on her when they are in danger, and countless people have received her blessing. Although Guan Yin is part of the Buddhist system, you don't need to be Buddhist to call upon her. You will still receive her unconditional love, her motherly love, her unconditional care, and her assistance.

Every religion, every belief system, has its own God or gods, but in fact there is only one God, one creator of the universe: the link between all religions, all spiritual teachings, is unconditional love. When you offer unconditional love, Buddhas will help you, Jesus and Mary will help you, healing angels will help you, Taoist saints will help you, the Jewish prophets will help you. Countless high spiritual beings will help you.

Millions of people love Jesus. He said, "Your sins are forgiven. You are healed," and miracles happened. What kind of healing techniques did Jesus use? He simply showed his unconditional love and forgiveness. He showed the power of the Divine, creating one miracle after another.

Mother, Guan Yin, Jesus — these examples show the power that can come from love, especially from unconditional love. They give us the deepest insight into healing, into blessing, into physical life and spiritual life: always offer unconditional love.

Say Hello with Love

When you get sick, do you complain to your organs and cells? *Oh, my stomach hurts. I'm really upset with my stupid stomach. I'm so tired, I've been working too hard, and now my back is so stiff and painful. I hate my back.* Stop complaining! It isn't going to make you feel better. It isn't going to help you heal. Turn your complaints into love and forgiveness. Why does the first sentence of Say Hello Healing end with *I love you?*

If you have back pain, say "hello" and use unconditional love: *Dear soul, mind, and body of my back, I really love you. You are suffering now. You have the power to heal yourself. Please do a good job. Something is causing your pain, but it doesn't matter what it is. I really love you unconditionally.* Then really give love to your back, just as you give love to your mother, to your true love, to your spiritual father, or to the Divine.

What does "unconditional love" mean? You give your love to others without any conditions. You do not expect or want anything in return for that love. Completely relax. Just give the thought, feeling, and message of "love" to your back. *I love my back. I love my back unconditionally. Love. Love. Love. Love. I have the power to heal my back. I have the power to heal my back. I have the power to heal my back. I have the power to heal my back. Love. Love. Love. Love.*

When you do this, close your eyes. Go into the emotion of love. Love carries incredible power. When you offer love from your heart, soul, mind, and body to your back unconditionally, the universe will help. The healing angels, saints, and Buddhas will see you offering unconditional love to heal your back, and they will respond. "Oh, how sweet this person is to practice love for healing. Let's help." They will send their light to your back, and you will receive additional blessing from them.

Unconditional love is a golden key to the universe. Just offer unconditional love, and it can help you heal yourself, others, and the universe. Love is not just a concept. It is a technique, a practical tool for healing. You will receive great benefits. Be patient and confident.

FORGIVENESS BRINGS PEACE

After love, forgiveness is another major key to healing. Forgiveness is powerful spiritual healing for all blockages — physical, emotional, mental, and spiritual. Forgive anyone who bothers you, harms you, or has a conflict with you. If you can offer unconditional forgiveness to those who hurt you, you will receive incredible healing blessings.

Why is this so? People who have hurt you leave an impression of that hurt on your soul, on your subconscious mind, and on the soul, mind, and body of your organs and cells. That impression will affect cellular vibration, causing the transformation between matter inside the cells and energy outside cells to go out of balance. This imbalance causes sickness. If you can offer the blessing of total, unconditional forgiveness to those who have hurt you, divine light and love will wash the impression of the hurt away. That is why forgiveness can heal existing sickness and why it can prevent sickness from occurring.

It is also vital to ask for forgiveness from those whom you have hurt. Unconditional forgiveness is easy to say but difficult to do. In chapter 5 I will give you practical techniques for applying it, in the Universal Meditation for Cleansing Karma. The more you can truly offer unconditional forgiveness, the more healing will happen immediately. The potential healing blessings are unlimited.

You don't have to take just my word for it. The physical and emotional benefits of forgiveness have been confirmed scientifically. Research indicates that forgiveness reduces stress caused by the unbalanced emotions of bitterness, anger, and fear. As an ancient Chinese sage said, "If you devote your life to seeking revenge, first dig two graves."

⁂

In 2003 I received the Universal Law of Universal Service from the Divine. It states:

A universal servant offers universal service. Universal service includes universal love, forgiveness, peace, healing, blessing, harmony, and enlightenment. If you offer little service, you will receive little blessing from the Divine, from the universe. If you offer more service, you will receive more blessing. If you offer unconditional service, you will receive unlimited blessing.

If you offer bad service, which includes killing, harming, taking advantage of others and complaining, you will learn lessons. If you offer a little bad service, you will learn a little lesson. If you offer more bad service, you will learn a more serious lesson. If you offer very bad service, you will learn a huge lesson.

This universal law is the golden key to healing, to life transformation, and to soul enlightenment. It applies to every soul of the universe. Your conscious and subconscious mind may not realize it, but your soul follows this spiritual law. It confirms the principle of offering as much good service as possible to the universe, including love, forgiveness, peace, healing, blessing, harmony, and enlightenment. Love will melt any blockage. Forgiveness brings peace. When you are peaceful, healing happens much more readily. When you receive healing, more blessing will follow.

When you deal with any situation, ask, "Am I choosing to offer service? Am I offering love and forgiveness? Healing and peace? Does my decision benefit others?" If the answers are "no," then you are not following the universal law. Stop and think. Use the wisdom you have gained. If you are thinking about doing something that doesn't fit this universal law, don't do it. Discipline yourself: "Okay, I will be careful. I won't go in that direction." If you can have this thought, this law of universal service in your heart, then balance and healing will come much faster.

Life will shine more and more. Universal peace, harmony, and enlightenment will come sooner. Bless everyone's physical and spiritual journeys. Bless the journey of universal enlightenment. Thank you. Thank you. Thank you.

Mind Over Matter

Over the last several decades, the power of the mind has become widely accepted and amply demonstrated scientifically. The importance of the mind for health and healing, and specifically the impact our emotions, attitudes, beliefs, expectations, and mindfulness have on our bodies, has been recognized by a new science of mind and body and is a driving force in the growth and acceptance of complementary and alternative methods of healing.

Because its methods are not in conflict with any other healing protocol, Soul Mind Body Medicine can complement any other healing approach. The revolutionary contribution of Soul Mind Body Medicine is its introduction of and emphasis on Soul Power, or *soul over matter*, as a powerful addition to the usual *mind over matter* approaches of mind-body medicine. The Mind Power techniques shared here are unique, and very powerful, because they are applied in conjunction with Soul Power. These techniques will help you develop the potential powers of both your left and right brain for healing.

When you consider that Albert Einstein probably used only 20 percent, perhaps 25 percent, of his brain cells, you will understand that the potential powers of the brain are unlimited. Learn the wisdom and practice the techniques presented in this chapter. Harness the great power of your mind. Use mind over matter to transform your life.

MIND POWER

Mind Power is the same as mind over matter, the mind's ability to make things happen, and using the power of the brain and of consciousness. Your mind can heal. Your mind can bless you. It has incredible potential to nourish every aspect of your life. Mind Power contains many facets, including intention, concentration and focus, imagination, flexibility, creativity, inspiration, and manifestation.

To understand Mind Power better, we can distinguish the power of the left brain from that of the right brain. The functions of the left brain include using logic and analysis, deduction and induction, memorization, calculation, planning and organization, speech, and language. The left brain supports your day-to-day physical life. It is logical, sequential, rational, analytical, objective, verbal, and detail-oriented. The right brain is responsible for aesthetics, creativity, inspiration, and other forms of "extraordinary" thinking and acting. It is feeling, random, intuitive, imaginative, symbolic, holistic, synthesizing, spatial, subjective, and nonverbal. The right brain, which houses your subconscious mind, represents and expresses the power of the soul. It receives messages from your soul. To develop Mind Power is to develop the potential of your right brain *and* your left brain — and also to balance, coordinate, and harmonize these two sides.

Scientists estimate that the human brain has about 15 billion cells and that over the course of your life, you typically use only 10 to 15 percent of them. In other words, the remaining 85 to 90 percent of your brain cells are dormant. This will give you a hint of the potential power within each of us. Awakening and developing these potential brain cells will be the major task for brain researchers in the twenty-first century.

The practices and exercises that I will share with you in this chapter will get you off to a great start.

The mind, which is the consciousness of the brain, can be divided between the conscious mind and the subconscious mind. The subconscious mind directs the conscious mind. Your conscious mind makes decisions, but it listens to your subconscious mind. To develop Mind Power is to develop both the subconscious mind and the conscious mind. While your conscious mind listens to your subconscious mind, your subconscious mind in turn generally listens to your soul. If all three are in harmony, you are in harmony — healthy, balanced, and happy. If your mind and soul are not in harmony, you will be ill or experience other kinds of obstacles.

You cannot develop the potential power of the brain through physical exercise. You have to use special methods of energy training and spiritual training. Soul Power, combined with meditation (Mind Power) and chanting (Sound Power), is the key to developing the potential powers of the brain, conscious mind, and subconscious mind.

This chapter will give you practical tools for developing the potential power of the brain and for applying Mind Power for healing. These exercises will help you to apply the power of the mind to heal, improve the quality of your life, and prolong your life.

FOCUSING THE POWER OF THE MIND

The mind has an amazing ability to focus, to concentrate, to condense its own power. Some masters can bend metal, such as a spoon or fork, simply by focusing. Of course, these masters went through serious training, and unfortunately a few frauds of this category do exist. But the capabilities of the true masters are an example of the potential that can be harnessed with the proper training.

Everyone's Mind Power differs because everyone's brain differs, and because everyone's training is different. But everyone's Mind Power can be increased tremendously through the practices I will share in this chapter. In fact, many of you may not recognize that you already have incredible Mind Power. This is often the case with scientists, doctors, teachers, and professors. They know they have good minds because of their affinity for research, even if they haven't had any special training for developing Mind Power. But most such people don't have a clue that they can use their Mind Power for healing — and very effectively.

The mind has so many capabilities, which are interrelated to various degrees. The wisdom and the practices that you will learn will benefit all aspects of your Mind Power — the left brain, the right brain, the conscious mind, and the subconscious mind. Soul Mind Body Medicine will also help you prevent degenerative changes in the brain, helping you maintain vitality and vibrancy for your brain and mind throughout your life.

FOCUS ON A VASE OF FLOWERS

Here is an exercise to help you increase your mind's focus. When practicing this exercise, do not wear contact lenses, since they may become dry and irritate your eyes. Also, do not do this exercise if you have inflammation of the eyes, swollen eyes, tumors in the eyes, glaucoma, or high blood pressure, because this exercise moves and concentrates energy to the eyes. However, if you have degenerative changes of the eye, farsightedness, nearsightedness, or macular degeneration, this is a perfect exercise for healing the eyes as well as boosting Mind Power.

Place a vase of flowers on a table in front of you. Sit down straight, facing the flowers. Here and in all subsequent exercises where I direct you to "sit down straight," you may sit in a chair or on a cushion or mat on the floor. If you are sitting in a chair, put your feet flat on the floor and do not cross your legs or ankles. Also, keep your back free and clear of the back of the chair. If you are sitting on the floor, cross your legs naturally or, even better, sit in the half-lotus or full-lotus position if you can (see figures 6 and

7, p. 53). Your hands can rest comfortably and naturally on your lap.

Keep your back straight. Put the tip of your tongue near, but not touching, the roof of your mouth. Try to keep your tongue in this position throughout the exercise. Contract your anus slightly. The placement of the tongue and the slight contraction of the anus are ways to promote the smooth flow of energy throughout your body, which is important for maximizing the benefits of the exercise.

Relax completely and open your eyes slightly. Grip your left thumb tightly with the fingers of your right hand and make a fist (see figure 1). Your right hand should grasp your left hand with 70 to 80 percent of your strength. Let the fingers of your left hand rest naturally on your right hand. Place this Yin/Yang Palm on your lower abdomen, just below your navel.

Let your gaze fall on the vase of flowers. While taking in everything in your field of vision, try to focus on the flowers without blinking. The longer you can stare, keeping your eyes open, the faster you will gain Mind Power.

This exercise is one of the simplest and most powerful ways to gain Mind Power. It will develop your ability to focus very rapidly. When you first attempt the exercise, you will probably not be able to keep your eyes open without blinking for even a minute. Just blink and start over. Force yourself to keep your eyes open until you can no longer tolerate the strain. Keep your eyes open *beyond* the point where you can no longer tolerate it. If you

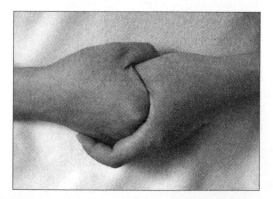

Figure 1.

Yin/yang palm

cannot, try again. The longer you can stare at the vase of flowers without blinking, the better.

When you continue to do this exercise, the vase of flowers may suddenly disappear. Do not be alarmed. It's a good sign that your Third Eye is responding. As you practice the exercise more, the vase of flowers will not only disappear, but it may be replaced by other things, perhaps a cup, a ball, a Buddha, or a healing angel. That is very advanced development.

It doesn't matter what images appear in place of the vase of flowers. Just do the exercise as long as you can. Start with five to ten minutes at a time, then expand your practice to a half hour, even to one hour or more. Do not attempt to practice for a half hour, much less a full hour, right away. Increase your practice time gradually, doing three to five minutes the first time, maybe ten minutes a week later, fifteen minutes two weeks later, and so on. Practice two to three times per day. When you practice, you must be relaxed. If you are upset, rushed, stressed, or emotional, do not practice this technique.

This exercise stimulates the focusing power of your mind. It activates all your brain cells. As you focus your intention on that vase of flowers, your brain cells can vibrate so dramatically that you feel heat in your head and eyes, or heaviness in your forehead. You may start tearing. You may get a headache very quickly, possibly a strong one. Generally speaking, this is no cause for alarm. A headache indicates that your Third Eye is reacting, vibrating, and opening. If your headache is really painful, use the One Hand Near, One Hand Far self-healing technique to relieve it (see chapter 7).

To further ground yourself, close your eyes to end the practice. Now, visualize the vase of flowers inside your lower abdomen. This will help move the excess energy from your brain to your lower abdomen, nourishing the Lower Dan Tian, a foundational energy center located there. Spend five minutes closing your practice by bringing your focus and intention down to your lower abdomen in this way. Your headache will diminish and, hopefully, disappear. If not, take a ten-minute break and then use the One Hand Near, One Hand Far technique again. If you still have a residual headache, do not worry; this is a reaction to the Third Eye opening.

This exercise is simple, but it is a very practical, profound, and secret training method for the power of intention and the power of focus. After a few days of this training, your healing power can increase dramatically, for both self-healing and healing others. If you practice this technique more, you can continue to increase your healing power tremendously.

FOCUS ON YOUR FINGERTIPS

Here is another exercise to help you develop the focusing power of your mind. As with the previous exercise, do not practice this if you have inflammation, swelling, or tumors in the eyes; glaucoma; or high blood pressure.

Sit down straight. Keep your back straight. Put the tip of your tongue near, but not touching, the roof of your mouth. Try to keep your tongue in this position throughout the exercise. Contract your anus slightly. Put both palms in the prayer position in front of your chest. Relax completely and open your eyes very slightly. Concentrate your field of vision on the tips of your middle fingers. Try not to blink. Keep this position as long as you can (see figure 2, p. 46).

Eventually, your fingers may appear to be expanding or lengthening. You may see them putting forth light. Instead of two palms, you may see four. The four palms could multiply further into eight or even sixteen palms. That would be great! The more palms you see, the more power you have developed. If you can see sixteen palms in a row, expanding outward from the center, you will have developed incredible Mind Power. Along with other extraordinary capabilities, you will be able to offer healing with just the gentlest of thoughts.

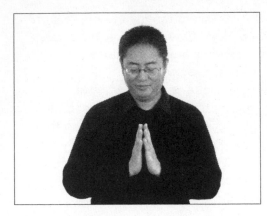

Figure 2.

Focus on your fingertips

As with the flower exercise, close by grounding yourself in your lower abdomen. The technique is a little different here. Grip your left thumb with your right palm and place this Yin/Yang Palm on your lower abdomen (see figure 1, p. 43). Bring your focus from your fingertips to your lower abdomen. Visualize a golden healing ball of light rotating counterclockwise there. Spend at least five minutes ending your practice in this way.

The flower and the fingertip exercises have been practiced for centuries. Training methods such as these have always been kept very secret. Historically, and even today, a master only teaches these techniques to a few very devoted and select disciples. I am honored to share them with you. Practice properly and receive the benefits. Remember to be gradual and patient. Do not rush. Do not force. Do not forget to close with a few minutes of grounding in the lower abdomen, because otherwise the practice can be overwhelming. You now have the tools to increase your focusing power, your healing power, and your manifestation power. The power of focus, of intention, of the mind is unlimited.

DEVELOPING THE POWER OF THE MIND

How can you develop the potential power of your mind? How can you stimulate the 85 to 90 percent of your brain cells that would otherwise lie dormant your entire life? Many people especially want to develop their right brain, which is in charge of creativity, inspiration, and spiritual capabilities such as the Third Eye. Here are two simple but powerful exercises for developing your entire brain.

NUMBER CODES
FOR THE LEFT AND RIGHT BRAIN

I would like to share a set of three codes that I introduced in my book *Power Healing*.[1] I learned these codes from my beloved master, Dr. Zhi Chen Guo. All you have to do is learn the codes and then chant them rapidly. You may chant aloud or silently. (If you are lying down, only chant silently. Chanting aloud when you are lying down will drain your energy.) This is such a simple practice. You can do it almost anywhere and anytime — when you are driving, walking, cooking, taking a shower, even watching TV. Of course, it is best if you can devote your full attention to the practice.

Let's start in a sitting position, in a chair or on the floor. Form a little "O" with your hands and fingers, with the tips of your thumbs almost touching and with the fingers of your right hand resting on the fingers of your left hand (see figure 3).

Chant the first code, the number sequence *01777, ling*

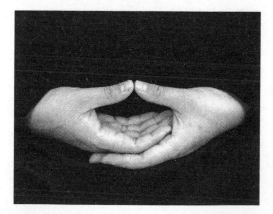

Figure 3.

Universal connection hand position

yao chi chi chi in Chinese (pronounced "ling yow chee chee chee"). *01777* is the secret code to stimulate the cells in the corpus callosum, the tissues between the left and right brain that transport messages between the two.

Then chant the second code, the number sequence *908, jiu ling ba* (pronounced "joe ling bah"), which stimulates the cells in the left brain.

Now chant the third code, *92244, jiu ar ar si si* (pronounced "joe ar ar sih sih"), which stimulates the cells in the right brain.

I recommend that you stimulate all the cells in your brain, left, right, and corpus callosum, by chanting all three codes in the following sequence: 01777-908, 01777-92244, 01777-908, 01777-92244. Chant as fast as you can, as much as you can. It will sound like this:

ling yow chee chee chee — joe ling bah
   ling yow chee chee chee — joe ar ar sih sih
ling yow chee chee chee — joe ling bah
   ling yow chee chee chee — joe ar ar sih sih

Initially, you can chant this whole sequence for a few minutes, but to develop the potential power of the brain, you need to practice for a half hour, one hour, even two or more hours daily. I greatly encourage you to practice for as long as you can. With devoted and extended practice, suddenly your Third Eye will open, or you will have some deep insights, such as, "Oh, I get it. I understand the secret of the spiritual journey, the purpose of life."

Almost any kind of meditation can help you develop the potential power of the mind. Chanting this sequence of number codes is one of the best ways. Remember to chant as fast as you can. Once in a while, slow down. Chanting quickly creates a yang vibration. Chanting slowly creates a yin vibration. These codes stimulate cellular vibration in the entire brain. They also help focus and concentrate energy in your brain. Always stay very relaxed as you chant.

Though I am sharing only a few techniques in this chapter, if you practice even just one of them diligently, you will receive incredible benefits. I encourage you to try these number codes. See how they serve you in developing the potential power of the mind and increasing your intelligence, capabilities, and healing and blessing power. These codes are a universal servant. I hope you will allow them to serve you well.

FAST IMAGES IN THE ABDOMEN

Mental acuity includes sensitivity and quickness. This Fast Images exercise is a great technique for developing the quickness (of reaction and thought) and sensitivity of your brain. In fact, it will benefit all of the many functions, and therefore the full potential power, of your brain.

Let me lead you in a guided meditation as a specific example of the Fast Images exercise. Sit down straight. Keep your back straight. Put the tip of your tongue near, but not touching, the roof of your mouth. Try to keep your tongue in this position throughout the exercise. Contract your anus slightly. Place your hands with one palm covering the other, with both palms facing your abdomen. Your thumbs cross each other. Your hands do not touch each other or your body (see figure 4). Close your eyes gently.

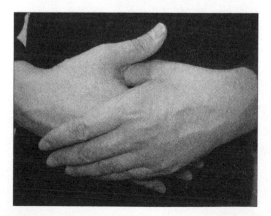

Figure 4.

Body Power for fast images

Think of your mother in your abdomen. (Always visualize whatever image or event I give you in your abdomen. I will explain why this is so important in chapter 5.) You love your mother. Recall how she raised you, educated you, and loves you. Right away, send your greatest love to your mother. Put any loved one in your abdomen — father, wife, husband, lover. As soon as you think of the person, send your light and love to the image in your abdomen. Go through your children, your sisters, your brothers quickly. Think about them at the same time, their personalities and other characteristics.

Continue to visualize in your abdomen. Imagine your best friends, one by one. Think about them. Connect with them. Doing so will enhance your relationships with them. If you think of them today, they may call you tomorrow. Now think about the sun, the moon, other stars. Say silently, *Dear soul, mind, and body of the Big Dipper, could you give me a blessing?* Suddenly — *boom!* — the stars of the Big Dipper shine in your abdomen. Millions of stars shine in your abdomen. All of Heaven is in your abdomen. All nine layers of Heaven, including the top layer of enlightened beings, are there. A beautiful temple, Heaven's dragons, Heaven's horses, Heaven's phoenix, Heaven's elephants, Heaven's birds, countless saints, countless Buddhas, and countless lotus flowers are all there in your abdomen. Receive healing, blessing, and nourishment from them all.

∾ଓଚଚ∾

Mind Power is a cornerstone of Soul Mind Body Medicine. Practice the exercises in this chapter to develop the potential power of your brain. Apply your Mind Power for greater healing. Achieve greater understanding, creativity, and insight. Improve the quality of your life. The power of the mind to heal and bless is unlimited.

CHAPTER 4

One-Minute Healing

We are now ready to apply Soul Power and Mind Power for healing. In this chapter, I will share a divine healing technique called One-Minute Healing. You can use it to heal any health condition of the physical, emotional, mental, and spiritual bodies. It is my gift to you.

You may ask, "How is it possible to heal in one minute?" since generally speaking, most healers takes fifteen to thirty minutes, and sometimes more, to serve a client. One-Minute Healing, which can remove energy and spiritual blockages instantly, works because it applies the power of *soul over matter* directly and powerfully. It can work for almost any health condition, although some cases may take several sessions before significant results can be achieved.

One-Minute Healing also uses Sound Power by invoking the most powerful healing mantras in history. A mantra is a special soul or spirit and also a formula of invocation, a spiritual gathering tool for healing and blessing. Throughout history, millions of people have chanted mantras. When you chant a mantra, all the souls who have ever chanted it will respond instantly by gathering together to bless your healing.

A mantra is also a special sound that stimulates cellular vibration of the body, organs, and tissues. It removes energy and spiritual blockages by promoting energy flow. The most powerful healing mantras carry divine love and light, which can remove blockages on the spot. That is why chanting mantras can bring about powerful, even miraculous healing results instantly. The essence of One-Minute Healing is to communicate with (say hello) and chant mantras to bring in divine love and light. The mantras and specific techniques are extremely simple, practical, powerful, and universal. They can transform your life.

BEFORE YOU BEGIN

You can practice One-Minute Healing in any position, anytime, anywhere. Depending on your environment and your condition, you can stand, sit, or lie down. If you'd like to do it standing, stand balanced with your feet shoulder-width apart. Bend your knees slightly. To do

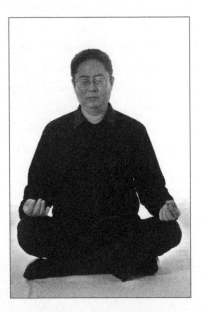

Figure 5.

Legs naturally crossed

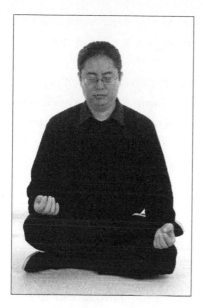

Figure 6.

Half-lotus

it sitting, if using a chair, sit comfortably with your feet on the floor. Keep your back straight, and do not lean against the back of the chair. If you are on the floor, sit with your legs simply crossed or, if you are able, in a half-lotus or full-lotus position (see figures 5, 6, 7). If you'd be more comfortable lying down, lie on your back or in any position

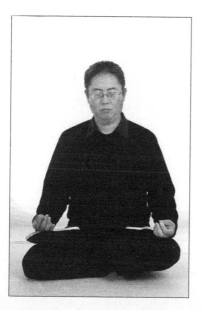

Figure 7.

Full lotus

that is comfortable. However, be sure to chant silently when you are in this position. Chanting out loud while you are lying down will drain your energy.

Next, drop your chin a little and place the tip of your tongue close to, but not touching, the roof of your mouth. Contract your anus slightly. Gently close your eyes and completely relax your soul, mind, and body.

Now we're ready to begin One-Minute Healing with the first mantra.

WENG AR HONG

Weng Ar Hong (pronounced "wung ar hohng") is one of the most powerful healing mantras from ancient China. Throughout history millions of people have received its healing and blessings, and it is still widely used today.

To practice One-Minute Healing using Weng Ar Hong, simply chant the mantra. The three syllables of the mantra have no literal meaning; they are simply powerful sounds for stimulating cellular vibration throughout your body. Specifically, *Weng* stimulates vibration of all the cells in the head. *Ar* stimulates cellular vibration in the chest. *Hong* stimulates cellular vibration in the abdomen. Together, all three sounds stimulate cellular vibration in all the internal organs.

Stand, sit, or lie down as described in the "Before You Begin" section above. Continue your preparation also as described above: Place the tip of your tongue close to, but not touching, the roof of your mouth. (Release your tongue from this position when you are ready to begin chanting.) Contract your anus slightly. Gently close your eyes and completely relax.

Also, hold your right hand, palm up, a few inches *above* the navel. Hold your left hand, palm up, a few inches *below* the navel (see figure 8, p. 55). If you have hypertension, glaucoma, pain, inflammation, or a tumor or cancer in the brain, eyes, or head, turn your right hand

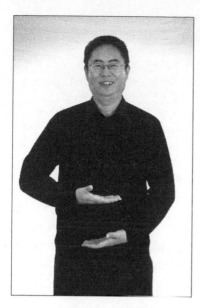

Figure 8.

Open San Jiao position

over so that the right palm faces down. The right hand is still held a few inches above the navel.

This hand position is called the Open San Jiao (three areas) Body Power position. Your hands should be close to, but not touching, your body to promote energy flow and healing. The same hand position applies whether you are standing, sitting, or lying down.

Next, say "hello" to Weng Ar Hong and request the healing you desire: *Dear soul, mind, and body of Weng Ar Hong, I love you and appreciate you. Please heal my* _____ [name your request]. *I am honored and blessed. Thank you.*

Inhale deeply and chant Weng Ar Hong in one long exhalation of three syllables. As you exhale and chant Weng, visualize bright *red* light shining in your head. As you continue to exhale and chant Ar, visualize bright *white* light shining in your chest. Finally, as you finish expelling the breath, chant Hong and visualize bright *blue* light shining in your abdomen. Inhale deeply once again and repeat the whole process for one minute. The practice of chanting Weng Ar Hong is summarized in table 1 on the next page.

Table 1. The Ancient Healing Mantra *Weng Ar Hong*			
Chant	Pronunciation	Area Stimulated	Color to Visualize in the Area
Weng	"wung"	head	red
Ar	"ar"	chest	white
Hong	"hohng"	abdomen	blue

Note that you can request healing for others as well as for yourself. For example, you can say: *Dear soul, mind, and body of Weng Ar Hong, I love you and appreciate you. Please heal my father's back* [for example]. *I am honored and blessed. Thank you.* Then practice for one minute, only this time visualize the colors in your *father's* body as you chant.

If you receive miraculous results instantly, you are blessed. If you are much better or only a little better, you are also blessed. Practice more. If no healing seems to have occurred, you are still blessed. Having no immediate or discernable results does not mean that these powerful healing tools are not serving you; it only means that you need to practice more.

THE SACRED HEALING NUMBER 3396815

The mantra 3396815 is a sacred healing number that my beloved spiritual master, Dr. Zhi Chen Guo, received from the Divine in 1974. While Master Guo was meditating one morning, he suddenly received a message giving him this sacred code and its significance for healing and blessing. He then awakened his third daughter and asked her to tune in to Heaven. She received exactly the same number: 3396815. The next day, they started teaching their students to chant 3396815 as a mantra for healing and blessing. Millions of people have since chanted this special number sequence, and many have received miraculous healing and blessings in every aspect of their lives. I am very honored to introduce this mantra to the West.

The mantra *3396815*, or *San San Jiu Liu Ba Yao Wu*, is pronounced "sahn sahn joe lew bah yow woo" in Mandarin Chinese. The sound of each number in 3396815 stimulates cellular vibration in a specific part of the body. Chanting *San San Jiu Liu Ba Yao Wu* stimulates the cells in these areas to vibrate in healthier patterns and frequencies. Table 2 shows the body area stimulated by each number sound of 3396815.[1]

Table 2. The Sacred Healing Number 3396815			
Number	Chinese Word	Pronunciation	Area Stimulated
3	san	"sahn"	chest, lungs
3	san	"sahn"	chest, lungs
9	jiu	"joe"	lower abdomen
6	liu	"lew"	sides, ribs
8	ba	"bah"	navel
1	yao	"yow"	head
5	wu	"woo"	stomach, spleen

The number sequence *San San Jiu Liu Ba Yao Wu* provides an inner massage to the body's organs and cells. It causes energy to flow in a specific circuit through the body. Starting from the chest (3, 3), energy radiates and moves down to the lower abdomen (9), across to the ribs (6), up through the navel area (8) to the head (1), and back down to the stomach (5). Repeatedly chanting 3396815 causes energy to flow continuously through the main organs and systems of your body in a healthy pattern, as shown in figure 9 on page 58.

The mantra 3396815 is a gift from the Divine (the Creator, the

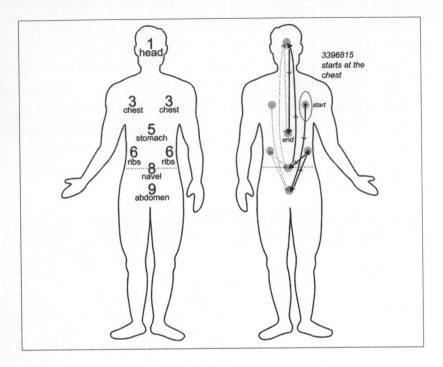

Figure 9. *3396815 stimulates different parts of the body*

Source, or the universe). This healing number is sacred because it unites the spiritual world and the physical world to support your healing. When you chant *San San Jiu Liu Ba Yao Wu*, you not only receive the physical benefits of its healthy vibrational pattern, but you also receive countless spiritual blessings from the universe. This mantra has tremendous spiritual power to gather light from the universe to heal and bless you.

The simplest and best way to practice One-Minute Healing with the mantra 3396815 is to combine it with Say Hello Healing. Just say "hello" to 3396815 and ask this powerful mantra for a healing blessing: *Dear soul, mind, and body of* San San Jiu Liu Ba Yao Wu, *I love you and appreciate you. Please give me a healing for* _____ [name your request]. *I am honored and blessed. Thank you.* You can request healing for others as well as for yourself. Then repeatedly chant *San San Jiu Liu Ba Yao Wu* as quickly as you can for one minute. You can chant silently or out loud.

The longer and the more often you chant, the better. You can chant many times a day, or even continuously for hours. You can chant while you are performing other activities, such as walking, driving, showering, exercising, cooking, or shopping. If you suffer from chronic pain or illness or from a life-threatening condition, chant as long as you can. The more you use this sacred healing number, the more it will remove the energy and spiritual blockages in your physical, emotional, mental, and spiritual bodies. Chant with confidence. Healing will occur.

SHA'S GOLDEN HEALING BALL

Sha's Golden Healing Ball, another special mantra, is a gift I received directly from the Divine on December 7, 1995. It is my great honor to share with you the message I received from God as I was meditating that morning:

> *I have created a spiritual gift — a golden healing ball to serve the universe in the twenty-first century. I give this gift to you first, but it is not for you alone. It is my gift to all.*
>
> *Because of your commitment to serving people through your healing work, I have entrusted this gift to you and named it "Sha's Golden Healing Ball." I choose you, Zhi Gang Sha, to share this gift with people everywhere.*
>
> *Tell the world that a golden healing ball exists in the Heavens and in the spiritual world. Tell people everywhere that it belongs to everyone who believes in it, who has faith, who has trust, and who is willing to use it. Healing will come to those who call upon this ball. Spread the message of Sha's Golden Healing Ball to people everywhere.*

Enlightened, I fell to my knees and bowed 108 times (once for each of the sublayers of Heaven) before God and the soul world, affirming: "With honor and pleasure do I accept this mission, and hereby pledge myself to bring Sha's Golden Healing Ball to the world. Thank you for making me the messenger of this great gift. Thank you! Thank you! Thank you!"[2] I have since shared the divine gift of Sha's Golden Healing Ball wherever I have gone, and hundreds of thousands of people have used it. It serves anyone who requests and applies its healing blessings.

Apply Sha's Golden Healing Ball for One-Minute Healing by sincerely communicating with this spiritual healing tool. Invoke its powers by talking to it in this way: *Dear soul, mind, and body of Sha's Golden Healing Ball, I love you and appreciate you. Please give me a healing blessing for my _____ [name your request]. Thank you.*

Chant *Sha's Golden Healing Ball, Sha's Golden Healing Ball, Sha's Golden Healing Ball...* continuously for one minute. If your Third Eye is open, you will be able to see Sha's Golden Healing Ball zooming instantly from Heaven to your body to rotate quickly in the affected area to remove the energy and spiritual blockages there. As with the other mantras in this chapter, you can use this technique to heal yourself and others.

Sha's Golden Healing Ball is a divine gift *and* a special mantra that you can apply anytime, anywhere. Its love, care, and compassion, as well as its healing power and blessings, are ready to serve you. Practice this One-Minute Healing method several times a day. Be sincere and persistent. Say "thank you" to Sha's Golden Healing Ball, the perfect gift from the Divine. Use it. Honor it. Benefit from it.

UNCONDITIONAL UNIVERSAL SERVICE

The mantra *Unconditional Universal Service* is an extension of a gift the Divine gave me in April 2003. This gift, the Universal Law of Universal Service, can be summarized as follows: *"I am a universal servant. You are a universal servant. Everyone and everything in the universe is a universal servant. A universal servant offers universal service, including universal love, forgiveness, peace, healing, blessing, harmony, and enlightenment. The more service you offer, the more blessings you receive."*

Eight months later, on December 4, 2003, I received further enlightenment on the use of this universal law as a healing mantra. At four o'clock on that day, I received the honor of a special blessing from the Divine. I was given an extraordinary new mantra for the twenty-first century: Unconditional Universal Service. This mantra, a major healing tool of Soul Mind Body Medicine, can be applied universally to serve healing in all aspects of life.

Chant this powerful mantra to offer unconditional universal service and to receive its healing blessings. As with all special mantras, the more you chant and offer service, the more blessings will come your way. Chant for as long as you can: *Unconditional Universal Service, Unconditional Universal Service, Unconditional Universal Service, Unconditional Universal Service . . .*

Unconditional Universal Service encompasses all seven aspects of the Universal Law of Universal Service, including universal love, forgiveness, peace, healing, blessing, harmony, and enlightenment, applied *unconditionally*.

What do I mean by Unconditional Universal Service? Think about God, Allah, Jesus, Mary, Universal Light, Guan Yin, Ar Mi Tuo Fuo, or any other spiritual beings you revere. Millions of people ask holy beings for their blessings and help. These highest spiritual masters serve you unconditionally, without asking for anything in return. They are pure universal servants who offer unconditional universal service. Although we may not have the same abilities, we can offer to serve humanity and the universe in the same way. We can offer our service by chanting *Unconditional Universal Service*.

Unconditional Universal Service is another golden key that will unlock any blockage and melt any obstacle in the universe. Each person will grasp the significance of this golden key according to his or her own spiritual understanding and awareness. The more you chant *Unconditional Universal Service* and offer service, the more blessings you will receive in every aspect of your physical, emotional, mental, and spiritual lives. Hold this key tenderly. Through it, you will receive immeasurable blessings. Serve the universe further by spreading this wisdom. World peace will happen sooner. Universal harmony and enlightenment will happen sooner.

Offering Unconditional Universal Service

You can offer Unconditional Universal Service simply by chanting the words. To serve others as well as possible, and to receive the greatest benefits yourself, love, compassion, and sincerity are important. Here are a few tips for applying this powerful mantra to heal yourself and others.

Offer Your Love and Compassion

How do you offer Unconditional Universal Service? Offer your pure love, forgiveness, healing, and blessing to everyone and everything by chanting *Unconditional Universal Service*. Offer service unconditionally without asking for anything in return.

Since everything in the universe is a universal servant, everyone's purpose is to serve to the best of his or her abilities. Look around, and you will see that everyone and everything would love to be of service. Some people help through charitable donations. Others give service by offering their time or skills.

Some people may say: *I don't have enough to offer. I don't have the resources or the abilities.* Others may think: *I am too tired and sick to help others. I can't even help myself.* Don't worry. The simplest way to offer service is to relax completely and chant the powerful mantras in this chapter sincerely. Chant *Unconditional Universal Service*. Through your thoughts and by the repetition of this special mantra, you are offering service. As you chant, you also receive the healing blessings of this special universal servant. The more service you offer, the more blessings you will receive.

You can apply the healing blessings of Unconditional Universal Service to any condition, illness, or problem, including unhealthy conditions at the physical, emotional, mental, and spiritual levels. You can apply these blessings to relationship problems, business conflicts, or to any other situations needing resolution.

The key is to continue to offer service even if you are ill or do not have much money or energy. Continue to give your love, care, and compassion to the universe by chanting powerful mantras such as Unconditional Universal Service, and many blessings will come your way.

Ask the Illness or Sick Organ to Offer Service

The same principle applies to your organs or illness. Though they may be ill, unbalanced, or not fully functioning, your organs and illness would also love to offer service. This is a very deep, little-known healing technique that is very powerful in practice.

Use Say Hello Healing to ask your organs or illness to offer unconditional universal service. Ask your organs to offer service by chanting a mantra. This powerful healing principle can be applied to any organ or body part that is sick or to any illness you may have.

For example, if you have a frozen right shoulder you can say: *Dear soul, mind, and body of my right shoulder, I love you and appreciate you. Could you offer universal service with me? Thank you.*

If you have any illness, ask the illness to offer service:

> *Dear soul, mind, and body of all my cancer cells...*
> *Dear soul, mind, and body of my sick lungs...*
> *Dear soul, mind, and body of my hepatitis C...*
> *Dear soul, mind, and body of my digestive system...*
>
> *I love you and appreciate you. Please offer Unconditional Universal Service, including universal love, forgiveness, peace, healing, blessing, harmony, and enlightenment. Please offer service by chanting with me. Thank you.*

Then continuously chant: *Unconditional Universal Service, Unconditional Universal Service, Unconditional Universal Service, Unconditional Universal Service...* Chant for one minute, but you can chant longer, even for a half hour or for many hours.

You are not asking for healing for your shoulder, cancer, lungs, hepatitis C, or digestive system. Instead, you are asking the soul, mind, and body of your body part or illness to offer universal service. The deepest spiritual wisdom lies in calling the illness, sick organ, or body part to offer universal service.

Give your love fully to the universe as you chant, and the light and love of the universe will radiate back on your illness or sick body part. The universe blesses you in return for the love you give. By giving service without asking for anything in return, you will receive incredible healing.

Healing Yourself

To practice *Unconditional Universal Service* to heal yourself, sit up straight, clear your mind, and be completely sincere as you say: *Dear soul, mind, and body of Unconditional Universal Service, I love you. Please give me a blessing to heal _____* [name your request]. *I am very honored and blessed. Thank you. Thank you. Thank you.* Then completely relax, and send your love, care, and compassion to the illness (or problem) and repeatedly chant: *Unconditional Universal Service, Unconditional Universal Service, Unconditional Universal Service, Unconditional Universal Service....*

Chant continuously for one minute or for as long as you want. Think wholeheartedly that you are well. As you chant, visualize the body part, condition, or situation being bathed in the golden light and healing blessings of the universe. Chant regularly.

Healing Others

Practice *Unconditional Universal Service* on your family members, loved ones, or anyone you wish to help. Direct its powerful healing blessings to help your friend with his liver cyst, your neighbor who has a weak heart, your sister who seems constantly depressed, your colleague who gets frequent migraine headaches, your son for his upcoming job interview — anything.

Point one hand at the person or situation you want to heal (or help) and start the healing by saying: *Dear soul, mind, and body of*

Unconditional Universal Service, I love you. Please heal this person. Bless his/her condition. Thank you. Thank you. Thank you. Then offer your wholehearted love, care, and compassion as you chant *Unconditional Universal Service.* Chant continuously for one minute.

If you can, I strongly encourage you to offer more service and gain greater benefits by chanting longer and more frequently. You can chant continuously for hours at a time or several times a day. The healing process may take days, weeks, or months. Be confident and patient.

Chanting and Healing Responses

Generally, chant as quickly as you can. Chant with sincerity, love, and compassion for all the souls in the universe. Chant out loud, quietly, or silently, but in such a way that the mantra bubbles forth in a continuous gentle murmur: *Unconditional Universal Service, Unconditional Universal Service, Unconditional Universal Service, Unconditional Universal Service...*

As you continue to chant, you or the recipient of the healing may feel warmth, tingling, or vibration in the area being healed. Some people's bodies may even start shaking in response to the healing that is occurring. Relax and remember that all such responses are a normal part of the healing process. If the sensations become too intense, try chanting slowly, quietly, or less often. Healing may be instantaneous, slow, or unnoticeable. Be confident and patient, and keep practicing.

&oOo&

The powerful mantras and gifts used in One-Minute Healing carry divine love and light. They gather high-level spirits to bless your healing. In one minute, your energy and spiritual blockages can be removed. You can heal instantly. These techniques, and some of the specific mantras, have been used successfully for thousands of years. They are my gift of service to you. Practice them. Benefit from them. May this sacred healing gift, One-Minute Healing, serve your healing well.

Thank you. Thank you. Thank you.

CHAPTER

5

Universal Meditation

For thousands of years, people have received great benefits from meditation. Scientific studies have demonstrated the efficacy of meditation for health and well-being. It has long been a vital tool for practitioners seeking to advance on their spiritual journeys. Many styles and kinds of meditation have developed around the world. Some meditation traditions require practitioners to visualize images. In others, practitioners strive to empty their minds. Still other practices combine meditation with chanting or require special body positions. I honor all of them.

With Soul Mind Body Medicine, I am introducing a breakthrough style of meditation called Universal Meditation, a powerful healing tool that can be used to deliver spiritual blessings to any aspect of your life. This kind of meditation involves creative visualization, within the practitioner's abdomen, of any and all images in the universe. As with every other technique of Soul Mind Body Medicine, *soul over matter*, or Soul Power, is an essential ingredient of Universal Meditation. There are two purposes in practicing Universal Meditation. The first is to serve your own healing. The second is to serve others — individuals, society, and the universe. If everyone were to apply the wisdom of Universal Meditation in their daily lives, healing, blessings, world peace, universal harmony, and enlightenment would come much sooner.

How does one receive healing benefits and spiritual blessing from Universal Meditation? Just say "hello." Simply ask the soul of anyone and anything you wish to connect with to come into your abdomen. As I will explain below, we place these images in the abdomen because that's where the foundational energy centers are. Call upon the healing angels, the Buddhas, the saints, the sun and moon, the trees, the mountains — anything you wish. Those souls *will* come into your abdomen. They *will* offer their healing power to serve your healing requests. At the same time, your love, care, and compassion will serve them. Universal Meditation is based on the concept that everyone and everything (animate or inanimate) has a soul and that everyone and everything has a loving and compassionate nature. Love and compassion serve all souls. For example, the sun serves the universe twenty-four hours a day, day in and day out. Similarly, the moon and the stars shine their light to the universe nonstop, trees exchange carbon dioxide for oxygen, and flowers give out fragrance constantly, without being asked and without expecting anything in return. They all offer unconditional service.

Every relationship is one of either harmony or disharmony. Universal Meditation teaches you how to be in harmony with all souls. You can use it to transform disharmony into harmony. You will learn how to put this into practice with the guided meditations later in this chapter. Universal Meditation will also accelerate the opening of your spiritual channels so that you can learn directly from the universe and the Divine.

STYLES OF MEDITATION

Millions of people worldwide meditate daily. Some practice well-known meditations that have been passed down through the centuries, while others concentrate on techniques for developing specific abilities. Although meditation is a personal experience, practitioners and researchers have long known the benefits of meditation on health and healing.

What is the secret behind meditation? The answer can be given in two words: creative visualization. However, *how* you practice creative visualization can make a world of difference. Whether a particular meditation originated in China, India, Tibet, North America, or anywhere else, it most likely will fall into one of two categories: *open-style* meditation or *closed-style* meditation.

Open-Style Meditation

In open-style meditation, the intention or focus of the mind is *outside* the body. Close your eyes and visualize the moon. Imagine the moon in the heavens among the stars. It is a beautiful full moon, and you can talk to it: *Dear soul, mind, and body of the moon, I love you. Could you give me a blessing? I am honored. Thank you so much.*

Continue visualizing the moon. Now it is so big and so close that it seems you can almost touch it. Feel the moon's light shining on your face and body. You are grateful for this nourishment from the moon.

In this example of open-style meditation, you visualized the moon, but its image remained outside your body; you did not bring the image inside it. In open-style meditation, you can use your mind's eye to visualize anything you like — a forest, an ocean, the sun, a bouquet of roses, a volcano erupting — but the images and visualizations stay outside you.

The advantage of open-style meditation is that it is very creative and active. You can visualize anything you want, but because the images are outside your body, this style of meditation does not build inner power very fast.

Closed-Style Meditation

In closed-style meditation, the mind is focused *inside* the body or on a specific part of the body. You visualize and focus on the body's five main energy centers, chakras, internal organs, systems, or cells.

For example, visualize your heart. Concentrate and see it beating with great vigor. Nourish it by bathing it in bright red light. All the heart tissues, muscles, compartments, and blood cells glow bright red. Chant to your heart: *Healthy heart, healthy heart, healthy heart...*

Because the images you are focusing on are inside your body, closed-style meditation develops inner energy faster than open-style. The disadvantage is that it is not a very flexible technique; it lacks creativity because there is a tendency to fixate on only one image. Creative thinking is much more powerful than logical thinking. Another problem is the dry-pot syndrome that can arise if you concentrate too much on a specific area. This is a phenomenon discovered by Taoist practitioners long ago as they concentrated on building the Lower Dan Tian, in the lower abdomen. If you focus your meditation excessively on a specific area, you will start to feel heat there. If you continue to focus on that organ or energy center, the heat can produce a dry, uncomfortable feeling akin to burning a dry pot. In extreme cases, this feeling will persist, even after you stop meditating. This indicates a serious imbalance of yin and yang and can lead to physical and other problems.

Open/Closed Style

Because open and closed styles of meditation both have their drawbacks, the best type of meditation combines both styles. It retains the advantages of each but avoids their disadvantages. I call this third kind of meditation the open/closed style.

The open/closed style of meditation is a very deep and advanced technique. The principle is to visualize images of nature and of the universe *within* specific areas of your body, such as the body's five main energy centers, the chakras, major internal organs, or wherever you need healing. This style of meditation is characteristic of Soul Mind Body Medicine.

Previously, we visualized the moon and the heart in separate meditations. When you focused on the image of the moon outside your body, you were practicing open-style meditation. When you concentrated *inside* your body on your heart, you were practicing closed-style meditation. You can combine these two examples to practice the open/closed style of meditation by visualizing the moon *in* your heart, nourishing and healing it.

Let me give you another example of open/closed meditation. This time you will visualize the sun in your abdomen. Close your eyes and say "hello" to the sun: *Dear soul, mind, and body of the sun, I love you. Could you come to my Snow Mountain Area? Shine your light and give me a blessing for my Snow Mountain Area. Thank you so much.* The Snow Mountain Area is a fist-sized energy center located in front of the base of the spine. Also known as the kundalini, it is a foundation energy center that nourishes the kidneys, the brain, and the Third Eye.

If your Third Eye is open, you will instantly see a bright golden sun shining over a mountain of snow inside your abdomen. Steam rises as the hot sunlight melts the snow. If your Third Eye is not open, just imagine a very hot sun melting a huge mountain of snow inside your abdomen. Visualize sunlight shining, radiating, and nourishing your Snow Mountain Area. Chant *sunlight, sunlight, sunlight, sunlight* ... for as long as you wish to receive the sun's blessing.

THINKING DURING MEDITATION

One of the biggest challenges for most people who are just starting out is concentration. The simple instruction to "stop thinking" is perhaps one of the most difficult for beginners to follow. The intent is to empty the mind. Many become discouraged and frustrated by the "monkey mind," the endless thoughts that crowd their heads as they try to meditate. However, if you struggle to stop thinking, you are not following a most important universal law, to "follow nature's way." If your mind needs to think, just let it think. After all, thought *is* a product of the mind.

Let me share a unique aspect of Universal Meditation that will change your view of thinking while meditating. In practicing, you will use your mind to create all kinds of images and place them in your abdomen. As you do this, many other thoughts will naturally occur, related or unrelated to the meditation. Do not worry. Treat every thought as a good thought.

If a "bad" thought comes to you, instantly transform its negativity. Use your logical mind to correct the thought immediately: *I apologize. I am sorry. That thought is incorrect. Please forgive me.* Then, lovingly place the thought in your abdomen. Do this for every thought that comes to your mind. Treat each one lovingly, with joy and appreciation, then place it in your abdomen. For example, if you are angry at someone, instantly say: *I am sorry. I will forgive you.* Do not let the anger bother you. Similarly, if you are sad about something, say: *I am sorry.* Let it go. Transform the negative thought on the spot.

If you have difficulty transforming your negative thoughts, immediately say "hello" and ask God's Light, the saints, Buddhas, and healing angels to help you. Whatever the outcome, do not be frustrated or upset with yourself. It may take some time to transform all your negative thoughts. Practice. Be patient. Your negative thoughts will diminish. When you achieve a peaceful, positive mind and are constantly filled with inner joy, you will be in a very special state.

You will find this technique to be a very powerful tool for training and calming your mind. Fewer and fewer thoughts will come to you as you continue to put the image of every thought into your abdomen. The better able you are to eliminate petty irritations and reduce your logical thoughts, the deeper the state of relaxation and calm you will achieve. Then you will more easily enter into the *empty* condition, a deep meditative state of stillness.

Emptiness is the transition point for unlocking all the secrets of Mind Power and Soul Power. Only after going through this door can your foundational power really get a boost, your subconscious mind and soul really start to develop in concert, and your Third Eye and other spiritual channels really start to open. The more emptiness you experience, the more benefits you will receive and the faster your spiritual capabilities will develop.

This is the real secret of meditation: turn off your logical mind and reach the condition of emptiness. The more you practice Universal Meditation, the more easily and quickly you can achieve this condition. Once through its door, you will have access to the infinite knowledge and blessings of the universe and the Divine.

UNIVERSAL MEDITATION: A BASIC EXERCISE

First let me lead you in a basic Universal Meditation. When we are done, I will explain the wisdom behind it.

Sit on the floor in the full-lotus or half-lotus position (see figures 6 and 7, p. 53), or with your legs crossed naturally. You may also sit in a chair. Be comfortable but keep your back straight.

Create the Yin/Yang Palm (see figure 1, p. 43.). Place the Yin/Yang Palm on your abdomen, below the navel. Place the tip of your tongue close to, but not touching, the roof of your mouth. Contract your anus slightly. Close your eyes partially and relax completely.

Remember that all the images you visualize during Universal Meditation are to be inside your abdomen. Imagine your abdomen containing the entire universe. Use your Third Eye, your inner eye or your mind's eye, to observe the images in your abdomen. If your Third Eye is not open, just imagine the images that I will guide you to see. Observe the universe inside your abdomen. Heaven is in there. The sun is there too, as are the moon and stars, Mother Earth, other planets, galaxies, and universes — everything.

Talk to the sun: *Dear soul, mind, and body of the sun, I love you. Thank you for your great contribution to the universe. Could you come into my abdomen and shine there and in the universe? Bless my abdomen and the entire universe. I cannot thank you enough.* See or imagine the sun shining in your abdomen. Enjoy its brilliant light and warmth. Chant *sunlight, sunlight, sunlight, sunlight...* for as long as you can. Imagine and feel your whole abdomen shining with sunlight. When you finish, thank the sun for its blessings: *Thank you. Thank you. Thank you.* Then say: *Gong song. Gong song. Gong song.* Pronounced "gōng sōng," these words mean "to respectfully and sincerely return." After finishing a meditation, it is spiritual courtesy to say "gong song" to all the saints and other souls who have come to give you their blessings.

Talk to the moon and the stars: *Dear soul, mind, and body of the moon and the stars, I love you. Please come into my abdomen and shine there. Continue to shine in the universe also. I cannot thank you enough for your great contribution to the universe. I am blessed and honored.* Then repeatedly chant *moonlight, moonlight, moonlight, moonlight...starlight, starlight, starlight, starlight...* for as long as you can. At the same time, visualize moonlight and starlight shining in your abdomen. Absorb the love, healing, and blessings radiating from the moon and the stars. Close by saying: *Thank you. Thank you. Thank you. Gong song. Gong song. Gong song.*

Talk to the Earth and invite all its members into your abdomen: *Dear soul, mind, and body of Mother Earth, all the animals, oceans, mountains, trees, flowers, rivers, I love you. Could you come into my abdomen? Give me and the universe a healing and a blessing. Thank you.* Then chant *Earth light, Earth light, Earth light, Earth light....* As you chant, visualize everything on Mother Earth shining its light into your abdomen. Close by saying: *Thank you. Thank you. Thank you. Gong song. Gong song. Gong song.*

Talk to the planets: *Dear soul, mind, and body of all the planets, I love you. Please come into my abdomen and give a blessing to me and the entire universe. I am honored, blessed, and most appreciative. Thank you.* Chant *planets' light, planets' light, planets' light, planets' light....* As you chant, visualize the light of all the planets shining in your abdomen, blessing you and the entire universe. Chant for as long as you can. When you finish, thank the planets for their blessing and light: *Thank you. Thank you. Thank you. Gong song. Gong song. Gong song.*

Talk to the galaxies: *Dear soul, mind, and body of all the galaxies, I love you. Could you come into my abdomen? Shine your light and give a blessing to my abdomen and all the galaxies. Thank you.* Then chant *galaxies' light, galaxies' light, galaxies' light, galaxies' light* ....As you chant, visualize the light of the galaxies shining in your abdomen and blessing you and the universe. Chant for as long as you can, and thank them when you finish: *Thank you. Thank you. Thank you. Gong song. Gong song. Gong song.*

Talk to the universes: *Dear soul, mind, and body of all the universes, could you come into my abdomen and shine your light? Bless my abdomen. Shine your light and bless all the universes.* Then chant *universal light, universal light, universal light, universal light.* ....Chant for as long as you can. After you finish chanting, thank every soul for its service: *Thank you. Thank you. Thank you. Gong song. Gong song. Gong song.*

So far, you have visualized and received the light and blessings of the heavens, planets, stars, galaxies, and universes. We also applied and received the light of Mother Earth. Next we will apply the light of the souls of those who no longer take physical form: *Dear soul, mind, and body of all healing angels; dear soul, mind, and body of all healing saints; dear soul, mind, and body of countless master healers and master teachers who are in the soul form or in the physical form, could you all come into my abdomen? Give a blessing to my abdomen and to the entire universe.* Close your eyes and chant *angels' light, angels' light, angels' light, angels' light...saints' light, saints' light, saints' light, saints' light...master healers' light, master healers' light, master healers' light, master healers' light...master teachers' light, master teachers' light, master teachers' light, master teachers' light....* Honor all the souls in your abdomen as you chant. At the end, thank them for their love, healing, and blessings: *Thank you. Thank you. Thank you. Gong song. Gong song. Gong song.*

In the exercise above, you visualized and imagined images of Heaven, Earth, and human beings and placed them in your abdomen. You requested their souls, minds, and bodies to bless your abdomen and, at the same time, to bless the entire universe.

In the introduction I quoted the ancient spiritual teachers, who made this renowned statement: *A human being is a small universe. All of nature is a big universe. What happens in the big universe also happens in the small universe. What happens in the small universe also happens in the big universe.* Well, your abdomen *is* the universe. The universe is one. The Divine is one. You, everyone, and everything are a part of the universe and a part of the Divine. We are all one.

As you practice Universal Meditation, you can connect with everyone and everything in the universe and request them to join you in your practice. Love everyone and everything in the universe unconditionally. Treat everyone equally. Serve everyone and everything in the universe according to the Universal Law of Universal Service:

I am a universal servant, you are a universal servant.
Everyone, everything in the universe is a universal servant.
A universal servant offers universal service, which includes universal love, forgiveness, peace, healing, blessing, harmony, and enlightenment.
The more universal service you offer, the more blessings you receive.
Offer universal service unconditionally, and you will receive immeasurable blessings from the universe.

Universal Meditation is an unconditional servant of the universe. Connect with this universal servant and practice. Receive the immeasurable blessings and benefits this universal servant brings: life transformation, soul enlightenment, world peace, universal harmony, and universal enlightenment.

PLACING IMAGES IN THE ABDOMEN

When we practice Universal Meditation, why do we deliberately place all our visualizations and images in the abdomen? The reason is that the fundamental energy centers of the body are in the lower abdomen. During Universal Meditation, we can remain grounded while building our foundational energy centers.

The abdomen is also one of the largest cavities of the body, so there is plentiful room to expand and receive benefits there. A significant portion of the body's blood is used in the abdomen, so Universal Meditation promotes blood circulation throughout the entire body. Although you *could* practice Universal Meditation in other parts of the body, it is best to do it in the abdomen.

The Foundational Energy Centers

One key reason that Universal Meditation is applied in the abdomen is that the two fundamental energy centers of the body, the Lower Dan Tian and the Snow Mountain Area, are located there. Both are storehouses of energy that must be replenished and expanded. Developing these two key energy centers will boost energy; increase stamina, vitality, and immunity; and prolong life.

The Lower Dan Tian is a fist-sized energy center, centered 1.5 *cun* below the navel and 2.5 *cun* inside the abdomen. (The *cun*, pronounced "tchuen," is a unit of measurement used in traditional Chinese medicine. One *cun* is defined as the width of the top joint of the thumb at its widest part. Although the absolute measurement of one *cun* varies from person to person, it is roughly equivalent to one inch.)

The Snow Mountain Area is at the base of the spine, in front of the tailbone. You can locate the middle of this fist-sized energy center by making a straight line from your navel to your back. Go two-thirds of the way along this line. Then go down 2.5 *cun*. This area is named for the snow mountain that Buddhists visualize there. This energy center is known to yogis as the kundalini, to Taoists as the Golden Urn, and to traditional Chinese medicine practitioners as the Ming Men Area, or the Gate of Life.

The Lower Dan Tian is the postnatal energy center of the body and also the seat of the soul. The Snow Mountain Area is the prenatal energy center of the body that connects with the energy of your ancestors. It supplies energy food for the kidneys, the brain, and the Third Eye. Both energy centers are vitally important for good health.

Forming a Golden "Dan"

In the basic Universal Meditation, you requested the light of the moon, stars, Earth, galaxies, trees, and flowers to come into your abdomen. The soul light of everything you placed there poured forth from the universe. The light of each soul and of each part of the universe has its own unique frequencies and qualities. As these soul lights interact in your abdomen, they stimulate, reflect, and reinforce one another, forming light of a new frequency that is proper and specific for you. This newly formed light will offer the right balance for your healing, growth, and development at the physical, emotional, mental, and spiritual levels.

The interaction and combination of the different lights increase their healing and blessing power. They join to form a golden light ball that, with further practice, condenses and concentrates further and further to form a lower *dan*, or concentrated, high-quality energy, which has its own soul, mind, and body. This light ball possesses incredible wisdom and capabilities for healing and blessing because it has gathered and condensed the essence of the entire universe.

Ancient Taoist teachings describe three *dans*, lower, middle, and upper. The Middle Dan Tian is in the middle of the chest and is also known as the heart chakra. The Upper Dan Tian is the Third Eye, which is in the center of the head. Taoist practitioners usually spend thirty to fifty years, or even an entire lifetime, building and developing these three *dans*. By practicing Universal Meditation, you can gather universal light into three light balls and place them in the three *dan tian* areas to accelerate their development into three golden *dans*.

With Universal Meditation, you could build a golden *dan* in your abdomen in a matter of months.

When the golden *dan* in the abdomen is fully developed, it contains the wisdom and essence of the entire universe. Now universal, this fully developed golden *dan* can turn into a living *dan*, which can travel to other universes to continue gathering wisdom and to gain greater capacity for service.

Why is it important to continue to gather new wisdom? The universe is changing every moment, producing new wisdom and knowledge in both the physical and the spiritual worlds. You can never learn enough; no one can ever acquire enough universal wisdom.

Heaven, Earth, and Human Beings Become One

The ancient Asian scriptures teach that the three major areas of the human body represent different parts of the universe. The area above the diaphragm represents Heaven. The area between the diaphragm and the navel represents human beings. The area between the navel and the genitals represents Mother Earth.

In our practice of Universal Meditation, our focus is on the abdomen, which represents both human beings and Earth. At the same time, our mind connects us to Heaven and the universe through the images we visualize. In this way, Heaven, human beings, and Earth are joined as one. As Lao Tzu, the ancient Taoist sage, wrote long ago in the *Tao Te Ching*:

> The Tao produces one.
> One produces two.
> Two produces three.
> Three produces all things.

Promoting energy flow and blood circulation in these three areas of the body promotes energy flow and blood circulation in every system, organ, and cell. This is a representation in the human body of the statement "three produces all things."

Your Abdomen Is the Universe

You do not need to walk a single step to find the Divine, for it resides right there in your abdomen. Lao Tzu wrote long ago, "Sit at home to understand the universe." Buddhists teach that "one grain of sand contains three thousand universes." With Universal Meditation, your abdomen is the universe.

Offer universal service and solve all your problems spiritually. If you can first find a spiritual solution for your physical-world problem, the physical-world solution will soon follow. Take the time to practice Universal Meditation. Some practitioners achieve miraculous results in just a few days. After a few sessions, your spiritual channels can open fully. You may suddenly see the vastness of the universe. For some, it may take weeks, months, or even years to reach that level of enlightenment. The path and time frame will be different for everyone. But you now have the key, the tools, and the knowledge. The more you practice, the more blessings you will receive.

PRACTICING UNIVERSAL MEDITATION

Before we explore applying Universal Meditation for healing and blessing, let me first explain some basic principles. Remember that every illness has its own soul, mind, and body. Say "hello." Talk to the soul, mind, and body of the illness or condition. Visualize it; then invite the illness to come and sit in your abdomen, as we did in the exercise above.

With the illness placed in your abdomen, think of anything in the universe that gives you pleasure and energy. See their images in your mind, and call them to come into your abdomen. You can call divine light, Buddhas, healing angels, healing saints, master healers, master teachers, the founder of your faith, your master, guru, or a special mentor.

Call on the most-renowned specialist in your country, a famous healer, your pastor or family doctor, your partner, a beloved pet, or even your deceased grandmother with whom you were very close.

You can call the sun, the moon, the stars, trees, flowers, oceans, animals, or a favorite hiking trail. Visualize and call anything you like to come into your abdomen. You can request healing from all kinds of images and souls, with one important exception: *Do not request healing blessings from a negative soul.*

If you do not follow this rule, you will pay the price. Ask for healing and blessings only from images and souls that are positive, loving, compassionate, pure, committed to service, and of the light. Respectfully ask all the images and souls you have called and placed in your abdomen to give a healing blessing for your illness or request: *Come into my abdomen and give me a healing blessing for the illness in my physical, emotional, mental, and spiritual bodies. Heal me. Thank you. Thank you. Thank you.*

After making your request, relax and meditate on the images you have placed in your abdomen. For example, feel the warmth of the sun and the wind lifting your hair. Remember happy days. See the love and happiness in a loved one's eyes, or enjoy the fragrance and beauty of a perfect rose. Float in calm ocean waters, feel the pleasure of a country walk, and experience the exhilaration of being young and strong. Let go of your worries. You have no problems. Be whole again. Start feeling and trusting your soul, heart, and mind again. Revel in the state of wellness. There is only universal light and love. Feel the golden liquid and golden light of the universe washing over you, within you, and through you. Visualize, truly feel and experience, all these blessings taking place in your abdomen.

You can expand the service of Universal Meditation beyond healing. Call the soul, mind, and body of every obstacle in your life to come into your abdomen. Think of all the blockages or conflicts in your relationships, business matters, and family dynamics. Then ask the universal light, the light shining from all the images and souls you wish to call, to come into your abdomen. Ask them to give a blessing for your problems, to transform the situations, to literally transform your life. At that moment, your life *can* be transformed.

In the rest of this chapter, I will give you guided meditations for nine specific and practical applications of Universal Meditation. These nine meditations were not created by logical thinking but by divine guidance. They flowed through my consciousness and out my mouth when I was in communication with the Divine Source and dictating this chapter. Repeat these exercises over and over. Healing, blessings, and life transformation will happen as you meditate — sometimes in the moment.

These guided meditations are for:

1. boosting energy, vitality, stamina, and immunity

2. healing yourself

3. healing others

4. group healing

5. remote healing

6. removing negativity

7. cleansing karma (removing spiritual blockages)

8. transforming your life

9. enlightening your soul

As you practice the Universal Meditations more, you will learn to use them for many different healing situations. I encourage you to be creative and flexible in your application of the healing tools I am offering you. Substitute, add, improvise, and change them. Healing does not have to be rigid and fixed. Understand the basic principles, then adjust accordingly, since everybody's healing needs are different and every healing situation is different. The energy of every healing is also different. Act confidently and be the healer you are. You have the tools!

Universal Meditation will serve you, your loved ones, society, and humanity. This universal flower remains open in all seasons. It never fades. It serves the universe unconditionally. Will it serve you?

Just as you must first taste the pear to know if it is sweet, you must try Universal Meditation before you know whether it will serve you. Taste first. Try first. Try several times before making up your mind. Many blessings will come your way.

UNIVERSAL MEDITATION FOR BOOSTING ENERGY, VITALITY, STAMINA, AND IMMUNITY

Let me guide you in a Universal Meditation for boosting your energy, increasing your vitality and stamina, and strengthening your immunity. The key is to build and develop the Lower Dan Tian, one of two foundational energy centers in the abdomen. This energy center supplies energy for all physical and mental functions of the body, so it needs to be replenished often. It is the key to long life. It is also the seat of the soul. When you build more foundational power, you will enjoy greater energy, vitality, stamina, and strengthened immunity.

We will be saying "hello" to and calling the light from the universe and the Divine to the golden light ball, your Lower Dan Tian, your organs, and so on. Speak with each on the level of the soul, mind, and body. Think of Universal Meditation as having a loving conversation with good friends.

To prepare for the following exercises, sit down straight. Sit on the floor in the full-lotus or half-lotus position (see figures 6 and 7, p. 53), or with your legs crossed naturally. You may also sit in a chair. Be comfortable, but keep your back straight, and do not lean back against the chair. Place the tip of your tongue close to, but not touching, the roof of your mouth. Contract your anus slightly. Close your eyes partially and relax completely.

Hold your hands together in the Yin/Yang Palm position (see figure 1, p. 43). Grip tightly, using about 80 percent of your maximum strength. Close your eyes and calm down as completely as possible. Then say "hello" aloud or silently.

BUILDING THE LOWER DAN TIAN

Dear soul, mind, and body of my Lower Dan Tian, I love you. You are the foundational energy center of my body. You are the key to immunity, stamina, and vitality. You are the key to long life. You are the seat of the soul. You are so important in my life. Please open your heart, mind, and soul to receive the blessings from the universe, from the Divine, from all the healing angels. At the same time, remember that you have the power to build yourself. Do a good job. Thank you. Now relax completely. If your Third Eye is open, observe the images in your abdomen: *Dear soul, mind, and body of divine light, I love you. Could you come into my abdomen and give me a blessing? I am blessed and honored. Thank you. Thank you. Thank you.*

FORMING A GOLDEN LIGHT BALL

Completely relax. Visualize divine light pouring into your body through every pore of your skin. See it moving through your muscles, tendons, organs, cells, and finally into your abdomen. A never-ending stream of light pours into your abdomen. . . . Light pours in constantly.

Divine light, from every direction, from every part of the universe, concentrates in your Lower Dan Tian to form a divine light ball, a beautiful golden divine light ball of universal light. . . . The ball shines golden light, shining, shining everywhere; it radiates golden light, radiating, radiating, shining, shining. . . . The golden light ball is vibrating, spinning, and shining, spinning and shining. Blessings from the golden light ball radiate to everything in your abdomen. How pure, powerful, and amazing this golden light ball is. The golden light ball shines brighter and brighter, this beautiful golden light ball, brightest golden ball. Shining, spinning, loving, blessing. . . .

Now the golden light ball transforms into a rainbow light ball. How beautiful this rainbow light ball is as it shines in your Lower Dan Tian. It is blessing your Lower Dan Tian. It is spinning in your Lower Dan Tian. Shining, blessing, spinning....

Now send this light ball farther and farther into the depths of your body — down into every cell. *Dear soul, mind, and body of the rainbow light ball, please send your light to every organ, every cell, every strand of DNA and of RNA in my body.* See the rainbow light ball spinning and radiating its light in every direction, to every part of your body. It is nourishing, giving power to and blessing every organ, every cell, every strand of DNA and of RNA in your body.

Now think of divine light again. Divine light pours in from the universe through every pore of your skin. As it flows through every organ, every cell of your body, it nourishes them, it purifies them, it heals them, it blesses them. Your entire body is divine golden light. Divine light from all directions concentrates in your Lower Dan Tian to form a golden light ball, forming, forming, forming into a golden light ball. More and more light shines. The ball gets brighter and brighter, heavier and heavier.... Divine light has formed a solid golden light ball in your Lower Dan Tian.

You may feel fullness, heaviness, tingling sensations, or movement in your abdomen. Or you may not feel much at all initially. If your Third Eye is open, you will see and experience some of these sensations.

The golden light ball shines brighter and brighter. You can feel your energy and power increasing. At this moment, you feel solid, grounded. You have incredible inner power. The more power you have, the more you continue to concentrate this golden healing ball. The golden healing ball is vibrating, turning, shining. Express your appreciation for the golden light ball: *I love you, golden light ball. I honor you, golden light ball. Thank you for the blessings you bring me.*

HEALING THE MAJOR ORGANS

After forming and concentrating the golden light ball, ask it to come in turn into each of your major organs and bless them. *Dear soul, mind, and body of the golden light ball, please come to my liver.* Then visualize or imagine the golden light ball flowing to your liver. Its golden light heals and blesses all the cells of your liver. *Thank you, golden light ball.*

Dear soul, mind, and body of the golden light ball, please come to my gallbladder and bless it. Thank you. Then visualize or imagine the golden light flowing instantly into your gallbladder. Give thanks to the golden light ball for its blessing.

Dear soul, mind, and body of the golden light ball, could you come into my heart? I am honored and blessed. Please give me a blessing. Then visualize or imagine the golden light ball moving straight into your heart and spinning. It spins healing, nourishment, and blessings to your heart. It actually turns your heart into a golden light ball. *Thank you. I am honored and blessed.*

Dear soul, mind, and body of the golden light ball, could you come into my small intestine? Thank you very much. Then visualize or imagine the light ball moving throughout your small intestine. It vibrates, heals, and blesses your small intestine. *Thank you. I am honored and blessed.*

Dear soul, mind, and body of the golden light ball, can you come into my spleen? Thank you. Visualize or imagine the golden light ball in your spleen as it starts to spin. Spinning faster and faster, the golden light ball clears all the blockages in your spleen and nourishes it. Your spleen is happy and appreciative. *Thank you. Thank you. Thank you.*

Dear soul, mind, and body of the golden light ball, can you come into my stomach? My stomach needs your blessing. I am most honored. Visualize the golden light ball moving to your stomach. Cradling the stomach tenderly and lovingly, it gives incredible love, care, compassion, and healing to it. It gives a blessing for good digestion and absorption. Your stomach is deeply appreciative. *Thank you. Thank you. Thank you.*

Dear soul, mind, and body of the golden light ball, could you come into my lungs? My lungs need your blessing. Then visualize or imagine the golden light ball instantly moving to both lungs and spinning quickly. In seconds, the golden light ball has cleared your lungs of blockage. Your lungs are blessed, moved, and deeply touched. *Thank you so much.*

Dear soul, mind, and body of the golden light ball, could you come to my large intestine to improve its function? Heal and bless my large intestine. Then visualize or imagine the golden light ball moving there. Spinning faster and faster, it gives incredible love and blessings to the large intestine, which is excited and honored to receive the blessings of the golden light ball. *Thank you. Thank you. Thank you.*

Dear soul, mind, and body of the golden light ball, could you come into my kidneys? Bless my kidneys. Thank you. Then visualize or imagine the golden light ball moving to your kidneys, where it resonates, blesses, and shines the brightest golden light. Your kidneys are most blessed.

Dear soul, mind, and body of the golden light ball, could you come to my bladder and bless it? Then visualize or imagine the golden light ball moving to the bladder and giving it a blessing of love. Your bladder is happy and grateful.

You have just asked the golden light ball to come to the ten major organs of your body. We started with the liver and gallbladder, which are the Wood organs of traditional Chinese medicine, and then moved through the heart and small intestine (the Fire organs), the spleen and stomach (the Earth organs), the lungs and large intestine (the Metal organs), and the kidneys and bladder (the Water organs).

According to traditional Chinese medicine, the Five Elements — Wood, Fire, Earth, Metal, and Water — make up the body and all things in the universe. The secret for good health is this energy flow: Wood → Fire → Earth → Metal → Water. Rotating the golden light ball in the organs of the Five Elements in this order promotes energy flow in the body's energy channels. The light of the universe nourishes, heals, and blesses these organs.

MULTIPLE SIMULTANEOUS HEALING

You can further apply Universal Meditation for Boosting Energy, Vitality, Stamina, and Immunity to any areas of your body that need healing, and you can do it for all the areas that need healing *simultaneously*. Here's how: *Dear soul, mind, and body of this divine golden light ball, could you go to my brain, spinal column, my right knee, my shoulders? Please divide into many balls, one ball for each body part I am requesting healing for, and give me a blessing for each request. I deeply appreciate all of you. Thank you.*

You can request healing for any and all body parts that are ailing. This golden light ball can be divided infinitely and instantly into many golden light balls. They can go to any number of organs simultaneously to bless all of them. The golden light balls are delighted to shine, spin, radiate in, and nourish any part of your body. When you are done, give them your appreciation. You have been deeply nourished and blessed.

CELLULAR HEALING

If you can apply the universal healing light to any organs or body parts, why can't you apply it to every cell? Well, you can: *Dear soul, mind, and body of the golden light ball, could you come into every cell of my body?* Then visualize every cell of your body being nourished by its own golden light ball. The balls are spinning, shining, and vibrating divine light in each cell. Every cell of your body is spinning a golden light ball; there are billions and trillions of them. Your entire body contains countless golden light balls. Practice Universal Meditation in your cells for as long as you want.

JOIN AS ONE WITH THE UNIVERSE

Tian ren he yi is a famous spiritual teaching from ancient times. It means "Heaven and human beings join as one." All the guided exercises in Universal Meditation in this chapter are examples of *tian ren he yi*.

Practice Universal Meditation for as long as you like. Keep the universal light and the golden light balls rotating, spinning, and shining in your body longer to receive greater blessings. When you decide to end the Universal Meditation, give thanks to the universe and the Divine for all the blessings they have brought you: *Thank you, soul, mind, and body of the divine light ball. Thank you, soul, mind, and body of the universal light ball. I am deeply honored and blessed. Thank you. Thank you. Thank you. Gong song. Gong song. Gong song.*

UNIVERSAL MEDITATION
FOR HEALING YOURSELF

In this section, I will give you examples of Universal Meditation for Healing Yourself. You can request any Buddha, holy person, Taoist saint, master healer or master teacher, Jesus, Mary, your spiritual leader, the best medical specialist you know, or your own soul to come sit in your abdomen to offer healing to any part of your body. You can ask the soul, mind, and body of certain acupuncture points, herbs, or procedures to heal you. These are just a few of the many tools of Universal Meditation that you can use for self-healing. Experiment and have fun with them. Practice and do a good job healing yourself.

To prepare for the following exercises, sit down straight. If you are too weak or tired to sit, lie down. Place the tip of your tongue close to, but not touching, the roof of your mouth. Contract your anus slightly. Relax your soul, mind, and body and close your eyes. Place your hands on your knees with your palms facing up.

THE SMALL PERSON IN YOUR ABDOMEN

Use your inner eye, your imagination, to look inside your abdomen. Visualize yourself sitting inside your abdomen, just as you are sitting now. Imagine that all of you fits there — from head to toe, from skin to bones. You are a small person inside your own abdomen. Feel the warmth and comfort of being enveloped by your abdomen. Sit calmly and serenely. A mini you, this small person includes your physical, emotional, mental, and spiritual bodies. In fact, this small person is your *soul*.

The secret of this meditation is to visualize the small person inside your abdomen being healed. *Heal the soul first; then healing of the mind and body will follow.* The following examples show how you can apply Universal Meditation for Healing Yourself to back pain, heart problems, stomachaches, and knee pain. However, the same general principles apply to whatever health condition you wish to heal.

SELF-HEALING LOWER BACK PAIN

To apply Universal Meditation to self-heal back pain, visualize or imagine yourself sitting in your abdomen as a small person. Focus on the lower back of your small person. Say to yourself: *Dear soul, mind, and body of my lower back, I love you. You have the power to heal yourself. Do a good job. Thank you.*

If your Third Eye is open, you can see the light changing and shining in your lower back. Healing is already taking place, but you can ask for more healing from anything in the universe. For example, you may love being in the forest. Why not ask the forest for healing? Just say: *Dear soul, mind, and body of a forest in the universe, could you come into my abdomen and heal my back? I am very honored and blessed. Thank you.* Be very calm, and visualize a beam of light from a forest flowing into the back of your small person. Feel the light, love, and energy of the forest pouring into your back. Feel the blockages melting away.

SELF-HEALING HEART PROBLEMS

To apply Universal Meditation to self-healing heart problems, visualize yourself sitting in your abdomen as a small person. Concentrate on the heart of your small person in your abdomen. Ask your heart to heal itself: *Dear soul, mind, and body of my heart, dear soul, mind, and body of my right atrium, right ventricle, left atrium, left ventricle, blood vessels, nerves, tissues, cells, I love you. You have the power to heal yourself. Do a good job. Thank you.*

Relax and open yourself. Experience and observe what happens. If your Third Eye is open, you will see changes occurring as your heart begins to heal itself. Next, ask for healing from the universe: *Dear soul, mind, and body of bright red light, I love you. Universal bright red light, come into my abdomen. Come and pour into my heart. Completely heal my heart. Thank you.*

Visualize beams of the brightest red light from the universe pouring into the heart of your small person in your abdomen. Feel your heart responding as you receive the healing blessings from the universal red light. Relax, receive, and heal.

In traditional Chinese medicine the color red is used in healing meditations for the heart because it has special healing properties for that organ. To complement the heart's healing, you can add another healing tool of Soul Mind Body Medicine: chanting. Create a healing chant of your own, or use the following: *Brightest red light heals my heart. Brightest red light heals my heart. Brightest red light heals my heart. Brightest red light heals my heart.*

Chant for as long as you like. Put all your love, care, and compassion into your chanting and send them to your small person and to your heart. Remain seated with your palms on your knees facing upward as you chant. Continue to see the small person in your abdomen glowing with universal red light. Your heart is being serenaded and bathed in the brightest red light. See your heart being happy, strong, and blessed. See all these things happening to the small person in your abdomen.

SELF-HEALING A STOMACHACHE

To apply Universal Meditation to healing a stomachache, visualize yourself sitting in your abdomen as a small person. Concentrate on the stomach of your small person, and ask it to heal itself: *Dear soul, mind, and body of my stomach, I love you. Could you help yourself? Could you heal yourself? Do a good job. Thank you.*

If your Third Eye is open, watch what happens to your small person. If it is not, visualize the stomach of your small person healing itself. Believe totally in the power of your stomach to heal itself. Encourage it and tell it to do a good job.

You can also invite all the brightest yellow lights in the universe to come into your abdomen and to give your stomach a healing blessing. In traditional Chinese medicine, the color yellow nourishes, strengthens, and balances the energy and function of the stomach. *Dear soul, mind, and body of the brightest yellow lights, I love you.*

Please come into my abdomen and give me a healing blessing. Thank you. Visualize beams of yellow light from the universe coming into the stomach of your small person, shining throughout your abdomen, and giving your stomach a healing blessing.

Another powerful technique is to visualize or imagine your stomach receiving a spiritual healing treatment. Although I use acupuncture in this example, you can apply the same principles to any physical treatment or procedure: *Dear soul, mind, and body of all the acupuncture points for a stomachache, I love you. You have the power to balance my stomach, heal my digestive system, and remove the blockages in my stomach. Could you offer healing for my stomachache? I am blessed and honored. Thank you.* Chant this mantra to yourself: *Acupuncture points, heal my stomachache; acupuncture points, heal my stomachache; acupuncture points, heal my stomachache; acupuncture points, heal my stomachache.*

At the same time, visualize your small person receiving an acupuncture treatment for a stomachache. Feel the needles as they enter your body and stimulate the acupuncture points for a stomachache. Feel your energy balancing and your stomachache disappear. This spiritual acupuncture treatment has some clear advantages over a physical treatment: 1) It is self-administered and 2) you don't have to know anything about the specific acupuncture points for a stomachache. The souls of the proper acupuncture points will respond to your request!

SELF-HEALING KNEE PAIN

To apply Universal Meditation to self-healing knee pain, visualize yourself sitting in your abdomen as a small person. Concentrate on the painful knee or, if both knees are painful, on one knee at a time.

Visualize your small person practicing the One Hand Near, One Hand Far healing technique on the painful knee. (See chapter 7 for specific healing applications of the One Hand Near, One Hand Far healing technique.) If the right knee is painful, visualize holding your right hand four to seven inches away from the right knee and pointing at it, while holding the left hand fifteen to twenty inches away from and facing the left knee. Chant *shi-yi, shi-yi* (the number eleven in Chinese), which stimulates cellular vibration in the knees. Imagine golden light flowing from the right knee to the left. Continue to visualize your small person performing self-healing inside your abdomen for at least three to five minutes. When you are done, give yourself a final message to get well: *Hao. Hao. Hao. Hao* (pronounced "how") is Chinese for "perfect" or "get well."

RECEIVE HEALING FROM THE SAINTS

In the last several guided Universal Meditations, you have been using the small person inside your abdomen to heal yourself. This technique is not limited to using your own soul for healing. You can also ask a Buddha or a saint to heal you. Just as you visualized or imagined your own soul sitting inside your abdomen, you can also invite a beloved saint to come and sit there. Doing so will bring you incredible blessings as you offer your hospitality to the saint.

For example, the new name given by the Divine to Guan Yin, the Goddess of Compassion, is Ling Hui Sheng Shi, which means "soul intelligence saint servant." You can say: *Dear soul, mind, and body of Ling Hui Sheng Shi, I love you. Thank you for your unconditional service and love. I invite you to come and sit in my abdomen to give me a healing blessing. Please heal my _____* [name your concerns]. *Thank you so much.*

Start chanting: *Ling Hui Sheng Shi, Ling Hui Sheng Shi, Ling Hui Sheng Shi, Ling Hui Sheng Shi....* Express your love of and devotion to Ling Hui Sheng Shi in your chanting. Chant for as long as you wish and offer your service to Ling Hui Sheng Shi. The longer you chant, the more blessings you will receive. When you are ready to end, give thanks and respectfully return Ling Hui Sheng Shi to the soul world: *Thank you. Thank you. Thank you. Gong song. Gong song. Gong song.*

If your Third Eye is open, you will clearly see Ling Hui Sheng Shi come and sit in your abdomen, blessing you on the spot. Even if your Third Eye is not open, you can visualize this powerful Buddha sitting in your abdomen blessing and healing. Some people react physically and may experience twitching, tingling, or heat in the body. Some people may feel nothing at all. Others may feel better right away, or their symptoms may only gradually improve. Whatever happens, or even if nothing happens, be grateful, patient, and confident. Ling Hui Sheng Shi loves you unconditionally and rewards those who are ready.

UNIVERSAL MEDITATION FOR HEALING OTHERS

To prepare for the following exercises, sit down straight. Sit on the floor in the full-lotus or half-lotus position (see figures 6 and 7, p. 53), or with your legs crossed naturally. You may also sit in a chair. Be comfortable, but keep your back straight, and do not lean back against the chair. Place the tip of your tongue close to, but not touching, the roof of your mouth. Contract your anus slightly. Close your eyes and relax.

When you are ready, think of the person to whom you would like to give a healing. The healing can be for any physical, emotional, mental, and spiritual problem. Say "hello" to the person: *Dear soul, mind, and body of* [name of the person], *I love you. Could you come and stay in my abdomen for a while?*

Visualize or imagine this person sitting comfortably inside your abdomen as a small being. Offer healing to this person by visualizing healing of the small person inside your abdomen. If your Third Eye is open, you will see the changes taking place instantly in the small person. Offer at least one minute, and preferably more, of focused healing. A few examples follow on how to apply Universal Meditation for Healing Others.

HEALING HEADACHE

If you want to heal someone's headache, focus your healing attention on the small person you have placed in your abdomen. Talk to the small person: *Dear soul, mind, and body of the head of* [name], *I love you. You have the power to heal yourself. Do a good job. Thank you.* Then think of a beam of rainbow light from the universe flowing through that person's head down to his or her feet. Boost the healing by chanting: *Rainbow light heals your head. Rainbow light heals your head. Rainbow light heals your head. Rainbow light heals your head.*

HEALING DEPRESSION

Suppose your loved one or friend is depressed, which, according to Soul Mind Body Medicine, is due to an energy blockage in the Message Center. The Message Center, or heart chakra, is a fist-sized energy center located in the middle of the chest. It is the key to one's spiritual development, specifically to communication with the universe. (See chapter 8 for a fuller description.)

Visualize or imagine the Message Center of the small person (your friend) in your abdomen. You will apply some powerful healing techniques to the small person's Message Center. Visualize bright golden light from the universe flowing through his or her Message Center down to the abdomen. At the same time, chant *sahn joe, sahn joe, sahn joe,* the pronunciation of the numbers three (*san*) and nine (*jiu*) in Chinese. *San* and *jin* stimulate cellular vibration in the chest and the lower abdomen, respectively. You can also chant: *Golden light flows down. Golden light flows down. Golden light flows down. Golden light flows down.*

Apply all these healing techniques simultaneously for at least one minute to heal your friend's depression. Offer frequent healings, since recovery from depression may take some time.

HEALING LIVER PROBLEMS

Call the soul, mind, and body of your friend who suffers from a liver problem, such as hepatitis. Visualize your friend as a small person inside your abdomen. Concentrate your healing on the small person with this special healing request: *Dear soul, mind, and body of the brightest green light in the universe, could you come into my abdomen and into my friend's liver to completely clear the blockages in his or her liver?*

Visualize the small person's liver shining the brightest green light and getting well. At the same time, chant with love and compassion: *Brightest green light, heal* [name]*'s liver. Brightest green light, heal* [name]*'s liver. Brightest green light, heal* [name]*'s liver. Brightest green light, heal* [name]*'s liver.* If your Third Eye is open, you will see the liver cells responding as they start to heal.

RECEIVE HEALING FROM THE UNIVERSE

In this exercise, you will call on the ocean to offer healing to others. You could also just as easily call on the sun, the moon, or your favorite rose bush. As before, call the soul, mind, and body of the person you are offering healing to and place him or her in your abdomen. See him or her as a small person inside you.

Ask for healing from the universe: *Dear soul, mind, and body of the ocean, I love you. Please come into my abdomen. You have incredible power to heal* [name of person]. *Could you wash him (her) clean, from head to toe, skin to bones? Completely wash through him (her). Clear all his (her) energy blockages and spiritual blockages.*

Visualize the universal light of clear ocean waters washing through and cleansing the small person inside your abdomen. Over and over, waves and oceans of universal light wash the small person clean. At the same time, chant a healing mantra: *Ocean water, clear his (her) soul, mind, and body. Ocean water, clear his (her) soul, mind, and body. Ocean water, clear his (her) soul, mind, and body. Ocean water, clear his (her) soul, mind, and body.*

All these Universal Meditations for Healing Others can be adapted easily for self-healing. Simply put or visualize yourself, your own small being or soul, in your abdomen. Be creative and have fun with Universal Meditation!

UNIVERSAL MEDITATION
FOR GROUP HEALING

To prepare for the following exercises, sit down straight. Sit on the floor in the full- or half-lotus position (see figures 6 and 7, p. 53), or with your legs crossed naturally. You may also sit in a chair or stand with your feet shoulder-width apart and knees bent slightly. Be comfortable, but keep your back straight, and do not lean back against the chair. Place the tip of your tongue close to, but not touching, the roof of your mouth. Contract your anus slightly. Close your eyes and relax.

In offering a *group healing*, it doesn't matter how many people are in the group with you. The same principles apply whether you do a group healing for five, fifty, or five thousand people. When you use

Universal Meditation in group healing, instead of placing one person in your abdomen, you can place as many people there as you wish and offer all of them healing. You can use this technique to heal many people at the same time, regardless of the different ailments they each may have.

First look at the group of people to whom you are offering a healing. Put the group in your mind and then invite them (silently) into your abdomen: *Dear soul, mind, and body of everybody in the group, could you all come into my Lower Dan Tian? Dear soul, mind, and body of everyone's systems, everyone's organs, and everyone's cells, I love you. You have the power to heal yourselves. Do a good job. Thank you.*

Visualize the soul light of the entire universe flowing through everyone in your abdomen. The universal *Ling Guang* (soul light) gives each person a healing blessing to clear the blockages in their systems, organs, and cells. Chant the healing blessing of *Ling Guang* for one minute: *Ling Guang, Ling Guang, Ling Guang, Ling Guang, soul light, soul light, soul light, soul light.*

Continue the group healing of all the small people in your abdomen with another healing visualization: *Dear soul, mind, and body of the golden liquid of the universe, I love you. Could you come into my abdomen and bless everyone? Wash everyone clean. Wash everyone's soul, mind, and body. Wash away their physical blockages. Wash away their spiritual blockages. I am honored, blessed, and appreciative. Thank you.*

Visualize golden liquid and golden light streaming from the universe into your abdomen and washing through everyone's soul, mind, and body. As the golden liquid washes them clean, chant for as long as you wish: *Golden liquid washes everyone's soul, mind, and body. Golden liquid washes everyone's soul, mind, and body. Golden liquid washes everyone's soul, mind, and body. Golden liquid washes everyone's soul, mind, and body.*

You have just learned the secret of Universal Meditation for Group Healing. Always remember to be flexible and creative. Practice. Millions of people are suffering; use your heart to serve and bless them. As more and more people learn how to offer group healing in this sacred way, world suffering will be reduced that much faster. We will achieve world peace that much sooner. I hope you will apply the wisdom and power of group healing as part of your service to the universe.

UNIVERSAL MEDITATION
FOR REMOTE HEALING

To prepare for the following exercises, sit on the floor in the full- or half-lotus position (see figures 6 and 7, p. 53), or with your legs crossed naturally. You may also sit in a chair. Be comfortable, but keep your back straight, and do not lean back against the chair. Place the tip of your tongue close to, but not touching, the roof of your mouth. Contract your anus slightly. Close your eyes and relax.

Remote or distant healing is offered in the same way as group healing. The only difference is that the person or group to whom you are offering healing is not physically there in front of you. For example, you can offer remote healing to a good friend who now lives abroad. You can offer it to everyone gathering for a family reunion that you cannot attend. You can offer healing to an individual or to a group of people, with no limitation on the size of the group. It works because you offer healing to the souls of the person or group whom you wish to heal.

To offer remote healing, think of the person or the group of people to whom you would like to offer healing. Visualize the person or group in your mind and place them in your abdomen as you talk to them: *Dear soul, mind, and body of* [name of person, persons, or group], *could you come into my abdomen? Let me offer you love and healing. Dear soul, mind, and body of the mantra Universal Love, can you offer your blessing to everyone in my abdomen? Serve them, heal them, and bless them. Thank you.* Then offer your love and compassion to them as you chant *universal love, universal love, universal love, universal love.*

As you chant, visualize universal love melting the blockages of the people you have placed in your abdomen. If your Third Eye is open, you will see incredible images as the blessing of universal love takes effect. Offer further healing by asking everyone to heal themselves: *Dear soul, mind, and body of everyone in my abdomen, I love you. You have the power to heal yourselves. Do a good job. Thank you.* Then repeatedly chant: *You have the power to heal yourselves. You have the power to heal yourself. You have the power to heal yourselves. You have the power to heal yourselves. Do a good job. Do a good job. Do a good job. Do a good job. Love, heal, thank you. Love, heal, thank you. Love, heal, thank you. Love, heal, thank you.*

Love, heal, thank you is a key mantra of Soul Mind Body Medicine. Remember to be flexible as you offer healing. Be creative. Offer remote healing to anybody or anything you wish, such as your pets, your garden, or your business. Teach this technique to others, so they too can offer remote healing.

UNIVERSAL MEDITATION
FOR REMOVING NEGATIVITY

Most of the examples of Universal Meditation presented thus far have focused on healing the physical body. But Universal Meditation is hardly limited to physical ailments. The remaining Universal Meditations in this chapter address the emotional, mental, and spiritual bodies and include your personal and work relationships. Use them as examples and inspiration to create your own Universal Meditations to bless any aspect of your life.

To prepare for the following exercises, sit on the floor in the full- or half-lotus position, or with your legs crossed naturally. You may also sit in a chair. Be comfortable, but keep your back straight, and do not lean back against the chair. Place the tip of your tongue close to, but not touching, the roof of your mouth. Contract your anus slightly. Close your eyes and relax.

Negativity can be defined as anything that is not loving, positive, helpful, or constructive. You can have negative thoughts, tendencies, or behavior. Negativity can show up in the form of irritation, greed, envy, or a whole list of other unhappy feelings. Perhaps you find yourself being mean, overly critical, impatient, or selfish. Perhaps you have been losing your temper, arguing with your partner, telling lies, or gambling incessantly. Negativity shows up in many ways.

Think of the negativities you would like to remove from your life. You can use Universal Meditation to work on them one by one. The technique is to call the negativity into your abdomen and transform it with love and light. Do it often enough, and you will transform your life.

HEALING JEALOUSY

You can call on jealousy, for example, to come and sit in your abdomen. Everything has a soul, including jealousy, even though it can be a very painful experience. Say out loud: *Dear soul, mind, and body of jealousy, could you come into my abdomen? I want you to turn to the light. You can do it. Dear healing angels, can you give me a blessing? Heal me of jealousy. Turn jealousy to the light. Remove jealousy from my heart, mind, and soul. I am blessed. Thank you.*

Visualize the body of jealousy sitting inside your abdomen. It might look like a glowering green monster. Invite the healing angels into your abdomen to shine their light and give a healing blessing. Invite other images and souls from the universe to also come into your abdomen to bless and transform the negativity you are working on. Repeatedly chant: *Healing angels' light. Healing angels' light. Healing angels' light. Healing angels' light. Love and light. Love and light. Love and light. Love and light.*

You can repeat this healing technique for each of the negativities you want to remove from your life. Create your own mantras for transforming negativity and chant them. Chant often and for as long as you like. Over time, you will find the negativities disappearing from your life. You will be happier, healthier, and a better soul.

The underlying wisdom here is that if someone is

successful, there are spiritual reasons. If someone is unsuccessful, there are also spiritual reasons. Almost everything significant that happens has a spiritual reason. If other people have success or other qualities that you are jealous of, understand that what they have achieved is a blessing from the Divine and the universe. Jealousy cannot help to improve anything in your life, so it is best just to get rid of it.

HEALING EGO

Another example of negativity is having too big an ego. You may be someone who continually thinks: *I am the best. No one is more perfect than me.* In some ways, this is the flip side of jealousy. What you have, what successes you achieve, are all blessings from the Divine and the universe. Those are the real reasons and real source of your successes. Do not be too proud of anything. Humbleness is vital for self-improvement.

If you have a big ego that you would like to work on, visualize yourself as a small person in the abdomen. Think that you are a universal servant, and tell yourself: *I am a universal servant. You are a universal servant. Everyone and everything is a universal servant. I am here to serve.* Reinforce the message by continually chanting: *universal servant, universal servant, universal servant, universal servant.* Chant for at least one minute. When you finish, thank the Divine and the universe for their blessings. Without these blessings, it would have been very hard to get to where you are today. Express your appreciation for another minute or longer: *Thank you. Thank you. Thank you. Thank you. I am blessed. I am blessed. I am blessed. I am blessed. I am honored. I am honored. I am honored. I am honored.* Gratitude is key to ensuring your continued success. Together, humbleness and gratitude are the keys to releasing the bonds of ego.

Because this is such an important practice, let me summarize how to use Universal Meditation for removing negativity:

- Call the negativities into your abdomen.
- Apply the love and light of the Divine and the universe to heal them.
- Chant *love and light*, the golden keys to removing negativity: *Love and light, love and light, love and light, love and light.*
- Thank the Divine and the universe: *Thank you. Thank you. Thank you.*

The power of love and light pours into the negativities you have placed in your abdomen, transforming them to light on the spot. May this Universal Meditation serve you well.

UNIVERSAL MEDITATION FOR CLEANSING KARMA

As discussed in chapter 1, the record of your service, of everything you have ever done to others and to the universe, is recorded permanently in the spiritual world. Good service such as expressing love, showing kindness, and helping others builds your virtue, good karma, or *te*. Bad service such as killing, cheating, and hurting others, or being angry or vengeful generates spiritual blockages and spiritual debt, which you carry as bad karma.

To review, virtue nourishes your soul, but bad karma harms your soul and blocks your journey. Bad karma is a spiritual blockage. When you die, your soul is judged based on the virtue and karma you have accumulated. The less bad karma your soul carries, the more fulfilled, happier, healthier, and easier your life will be. This is true not only for your present life but also for your future lives. Your karma will also affect the lives of your descendants.

You can do something about the bad karma you carry by cleansing it. Universal Meditation gives you a secret tool for cleansing karma — both your own and that of others. Some people experience a miraculous healing or life blessing after practicing Universal Meditation for Cleansing Karma. Others may require numerous sessions before they feel or notice any significant results. As with all spiritual tools of Soul Mind Body Medicine, be sincere, grateful, and have no expectations.

To prepare for the following exercises, sit on the floor in the full- or half-lotus position, or with your legs crossed naturally. You may also sit in a chair. Be comfortable, but keep your back straight. Place the tip of your tongue close to, but not touching, the roof of your mouth. Contract your anus slightly. Close your eyes and relax.

ASK FOR FORGIVENESS

Loving forgiveness is the key to cleansing karma. The two aspects of this secret wisdom are being forgiven and forgiving others. Let's start with asking for forgiveness from others.

Ask for forgiveness from others, sincerely and humbly. Start by visualizing all the souls you have ever hurt, consciously or unconsciously. Call them and place them inside your abdomen: *Dear soul, mind, and body of everyone and everything I have ever hurt, harmed, or taken advantage of in this lifetime or in past lifetimes, could you come into my abdomen? I love you. I sincerely ask you to forgive me for all my mistakes in all my lifetimes. Please forgive me. I am sorry.*

Ask divine light to come into your abdomen and bless the forgiveness that these souls extend to you. Chant to receive the blessing of God's light: *God's light, God's light, God's light, God's light* or *divine light, divine light, divine light, divine light* or *universal light, universal light, universal light, universal light.* Ask the light to bless you and everyone you have hurt. Chant continuously for at least one minute. When you are done, thank the light and all the souls for their love and blessings. Then respectfully send the spirits and souls back: *Thank you. Thank you. Thank you. Gong song. Gong song. Gong song.*

Depending on your level of sincerity and honesty, many of the souls you have called into your abdomen may forgive you. If you receive their forgiveness, you are blessed. The more souls who forgive you, the better the healing results you can achieve. If some souls will not forgive you this time, it doesn't mean they never will. You need to do more. Perhaps you need to ask for forgiveness again. Perhaps you need to offer more service or pay off more of your karmic debt.

If you made a big mistake, caused terrible pain, or were maybe even involved with killing, merely asking for forgiveness may not be enough. You may need to give the soul you have harmed some of your good virtue, which is the record of your good service. How can you give your virtue to others? Simply ask the Divine and the spiritual world to transfer some of the good karma from your virtue bank to the souls to whom you are indebted. You can say, "Dear God, give my good virtue to this person."

After you return your virtue to someone, you may experience even greater struggles in your life. Heartbreak, illness, bankruptcy, failures — all kinds of things can happen. You have to suffer physically, emotionally, mentally, and spiritually in order to cleanse your karma. Struggles, pain, and difficulties are all part of the process of cleansing karma. They cannot be avoided. If not in this life, then in the next, you must return your virtue to the souls you owe. Spiritual law is serious. Karma cannot be wiped clean. It must be repaid.

FORGIVE OTHERS

The second aspect of cleansing karma is to forgive those who are indebted to you. Visualize all the souls who need your forgiveness, and call them into your abdomen: *Dear soul, mind, body of everyone and everything who has ever hurt me, taken advantage of me, or harmed me throughout my lifetimes, could you come into my abdomen? I love you. I totally forgive you. You do not have to return anything to me.*

Then, forgive all the souls who have ever hurt you. Completely and unconditionally forgive them. This is absolutely vital for cleansing your karma. Do not just say the words. Truly offer your forgiveness. As you forgive, ask for and receive the blessing of the Divine by chanting *God's light* or *universal light*. Chant for at least one minute or, preferably, for much longer.

In unconditionally forgiving others, never think you have lost out or been taken advantage of. If you offer some service that greatly benefits someone or society as a whole, you may not get returns from the material world in the form of money or property, but you will receive incredible spiritual blessings. For example, you may recover from a serious illness or injury; your relationships will seem blessed; your business will run smoothly; you will be healthier and live longer; disasters will be averted, and many other blessings will come into your life.

Heaven Is Most Fair

As we saw in chapter 1, a very famous ancient Chinese saying best summarizes the principles I have just explained: *Heaven is most fair.* Heaven has a record of everything in your life. Heaven knows all your mistakes and good deeds, knows any recompensing efforts you make, especially unconditional forgiveness. After you have made amends, one day, unbeknownst to you, the Divine and Heaven will give you a multitude of blessings. Only later will you realize what great blessings you were given.

Remember, success and disaster happen at the same time. When disaster comes, it clears your karma further. Disaster or blockages will not end until all your karma is cleared, but it may take a long time, perhaps years or several lifetimes. However, as you work on be-coming karma free, fewer disasters will affect you and more blessings will shower your life.

Universal Service Is Required

The Universal Meditation for Cleansing Karma gives you two practi-cal tools for cleansing your karma: asking forgiveness from those you have hurt, and forgiving those who have hurt you. These two aspects of forgiveness must be applied unconditionally in order to cleanse your karma. Practice these two aspects of forgiveness often. Though clearing karma is a gradual process that may take years or even life-times (after all, you have accumulated your karma over lifetimes), the rewards are immeasurable. Unconditional forgiveness will bring healing and unlimited blessings into every aspect of your life.

Keep in mind that you must also follow the Universal Law of Universal Service (see chapter 2) to cleanse your karma, heal, and re-ceive blessings. Always offer unconditional universal service, includ-ing universal love, forgiveness, peace, healing, blessing, harmony, and enlightenment. Do not complain, and have no attachment. Fol-low these simple rules and use the tools I have given you. Together, they are the most practical and direct way for you to cleanse your karma, improve your life, and bless your journey.

UNIVERSAL MEDITATION
FOR LIFE TRANSFORMATION

The purpose of using Universal Meditation for life transformation is to purify one's soul, mind, and body to live a more fulfilled and mean-ingful life. Taoists liken the process to transforming ore into gold. One collects and discards the slag and scum to purify the gold. This is a continuous process in which each successive clearing produces a purer product until, ultimately, the "gold pill" is produced. For those on the spiritual journey, life transformation involves transforming the soul (enlightenment), transforming the mind (purity of mind), and transforming the body (eternal body).

On a day-to-day level, life transformation is about purifying your life so that it can be filled with more divine light and love. You have the power to transform any aspect of your life — health, business, relationships, conflicts — into a more loving and harmonious state. Healing will follow as a result.

To prepare for each of the following exercises, sit on the floor in the full-lotus or half-lotus position, or with your legs crossed naturally. You may also sit in a chair. Be comfortable, but keep your back straight, and do not lean back against the chair. Place the tip of your tongue close to, but not touching, the roof of your mouth. Contract your anus slightly. Close your eyes and relax.

TRANSFORMING RELATIONSHIPS

Let me give an example of life transformation in relationships. If you have a problem with your loved one or partner, you can help resolve it with Universal Meditation.

Visualize and call your partner into your abdomen and discuss the problem with his or her small person that you have placed there: *Dear soul, mind, and body of* _____ [name of person], *could you come into my abdomen? I love you. We have a problem. Let's talk about it. This is how I see the situation. You see it another way. How can we resolve the situation? Let's meet in the middle. Let's both take more responsibility for the problem and for fixing it.*

Look at the situation together and talk it out, all as a visualization inside your abdomen. First, try to understand the part you play. Perhaps you did or said something that contributed. If you had said things differently or reacted differently, perhaps the problem could have been avoided. Find your own weaknesses. Own up to improper actions and behavior. Apologize for your mistakes. Do all this with love and forgiveness. Then harmony and resolution will come about much faster. Be sure not to complain about each other. As you continue your visualization, have both of you take responsibility for your actions. Ask the universe to bless your relationship. Ask that love, forgiveness, and harmony bless the two of you.

Chant repeatedly: *We forgive each other. We forgive each other. We forgive each other. We forgive each other. We understand each other. We cooperate with each other. We both take responsibility for the problem and the solution.* Then chant *love, peace, and harmony, love, peace, and harmony, love, peace, and harmony, love, peace, and harmony* for one minute or longer. As you chant, visualize the light of love, peace, harmony, and forgiveness blessing the two of you within your abdomen.

Use this Universal Meditation for Life Transformation as a spiritual tool to resolve your relationship problems — in the abdomen. It may sound incredible and improbable, even impossible, but give it a try!

TRANSFORMING THE CORPORATE WORLD

In this exercise we will use Universal Meditation for the life transformation of a business or for matters in the corporate world. Let's suppose your company has a complex problem that your work team needs to solve. Hold a soul meeting in your abdomen! Visualize and call the souls of all your team members into your abdomen. See your own small person in your abdomen with your fellow team members. Start the meeting by inviting every soul attending to chant, offer universal service, and receive blessings from the universe with you. Chant continuously: *universal service, universal service, universal service, universal service; God's light, God's light, God's light, God's light.* Chanting "universal service" reminds all present of their purpose. Ultimately, universal service is the purpose of your team and of your business; it is everyone's purpose.

After chanting, ask the team members in your abdomen to be supportive of each other and to cooperate on the soul level. Then open the floor to discussion. Explore and analyze the situation. Ask for everyone's input. Discuss solutions, and then come up with a working plan. Before you end the meeting, ask every soul of your team for his or her full participation and blessing of the solution. This is to facilitate smooth real-world execution of the resolutions adopted at your soul meeting.

You can similarly hold soul meetings in your abdomen for business planning, brainstorming, launching new initiatives, developing marketing plans, strategizing, and more. Try it. Hold your own soul meetings and watch the spiritual solutions you have developed manifest in the real world. Conduct your soul meetings before actual physical meetings for greater cooperation, harmony, and successful outcomes.

Remember, all businesses or corporations have two teams: the physical-world team and the spiritual world or Heaven's team. Both have to join hands and work in harmony for the company to be successful. Help make it happen by holding a soul meeting in your abdomen with both business teams. After you have called your physical-world business team into your abdomen, be sure also to ask your heavenly business team to come and give guidance on the spiritual level. The solutions you develop together will be the ones that can be implemented most successfully in the physical world. As you end your meeting, ask for the blessing of your Heaven's team for the resolutions adopted and for every aspect of your business.

During the act of meditation much wisdom can be transferred to you from the Divine and from the universe. If your spiritual channels are open, you can receive incredible guidance from your Heaven's team. If your spiritual channels are not open, blessings from your Heaven's team will direct your mind to coordinate with them. Afterward, you will plan, organize, and operate your business much more successfully. Remember that you can plan as much as you like, but success depends on Heaven and is much easier to achieve when you have Heaven's guidance and support.

Life transformation can happen in any part of your life you wish to change. You can help make it happen with Universal Meditation by holding a soul meeting in your abdomen. Change family dynamics, harmonize your relationship with your partner, negotiate a better job, manage your business better. You can transform any problem, situation, or conflict and, in the process, transform and purify your life.

UNIVERSAL MEDITATION
FOR SOUL ENLIGHTENMENT

What is the goal of soul enlightenment? To purify ourselves. To stop the process of reincarnation. To become an enlightened immortal being to serve the universe. Buddhists believe that being human is to suffer and that enlightenment is the key to end all suffering. When one dies, the soul returns to the universe and subsequently reincarnates, coming back down to Earth within a few years for another lifetime of lessons, suffering, and, ideally, service. Up, down, up, down, up, down, up, down — the cycle of reincarnation goes on and on until the soul reaches a high enough level of purity to be enlightened.

To be enlightened is to have your soul's spiritual standing reach the ninth, or highest, level of Heaven. There are many souls at the lower levels, but progressively fewer souls at the higher ones. Each successively higher level requires greater purity, commitment, and service. If your soul is already at level nine, you have received many blessings and are enlightened. At this level, your soul can stop reincarnating; it does not have to come back to Earth unless it wishes to do so or is sent back for a special mission. However, being an enlightened being does not mean your soul journey is complete. Each of the nine levels of Heaven has twelve sublevels, so your soul would still have to ascend these twelve steps before completing its soul journey. That process can take thousands of years and many lifetimes. Persevere, and you will be like the lotus flower emerging pure and beautiful from the mud.

Life on Earth, a place of "red dust," is messy and dirty. There are many temptations. War, greed, poverty, and abuse are all around us. Disagreements abound, feelings are hurt, and lies and fraud are rampant. Bad karma is constantly being created. Soul enlightenment is a very difficult process for us human beings. It takes lots of effort and service to remove negativity; cleanse our karma; purify our souls, minds, and bodies; and transform our lives. Universal Meditation for Soul Enlightenment combines all these aspects to help you reach soul enlightenment faster.

Sit on the floor in the full- or half-lotus position, or with your legs crossed naturally. You may also sit in a chair. Be comfortable, but keep your back straight, and do not lean back against the chair. Place the tip of your tongue close to, but not touching, the roof of your mouth. Contract your anus slightly. Close your eyes and relax.

Visualize your soul as a small person inside your abdomen. Your soul is sitting there happy and content. Ask the special healing and blessing mantra, 3396815, *San San Jiu Liu Ba Yao Wu* (pronounced "sahn sahn joe lew bah yow woo"; see p. 56) and Sha's Golden Healing Ball (see p. 59) to come to your soul. Chant *San San Jiu Liu Ba Yao Wu* as quickly as you can. Ask Sha's Golden Healing Ball to shine pure golden light to purify your soul. Then ask these two special spiritual gifts to come and purify, in turn, your heart, mind, systems, organs, and cells. These two special gifts can give you extraordinary blessings, remove your bad karma, remove negativity, give you healing, transform your life, and greatly help to purify your soul, heart, mind, and body.

Use these two gifts on every cell of your body. Talk to your body: *Dear soul, mind, and body of my abdomen, I love you. Dear soul, mind, and body of* San San Jiu Liu Ba Yao Wu *and Sha's Golden Healing Ball, I love you. Could you come into my abdomen? Dear soul, mind, and body of every system, every organ, and every cell of my body, I love you. Could you all work together to heal, purify, and transform every cell of my body? Transform every aspect of my life. Please give me a blessing for pure love and unconditional service.*

Chant *love and light, love and light, love and light, love and light, unconditional service, unconditional service, unconditional service, uncon-ditional service* continuously. Concentrate and chant for at least five minutes. Practicing this technique a few times per day can give you unlimited blessings to advance your soul enlightenment. Practice consistently, the more frequently the better.

On the spiritual journey, those seeking soul enlightenment will be given tests from the spiritual world. Tests can appear in many forms. You may feel confused, have doubts, or feel emotionally unbalanced. Your body may shake, or you could feel an internal trembling. Friends and family may desert you. Do not think that anything is wrong. These are all normal reactions, all part of the process of soul cleansing and purification. Spiritual testing and physical reactions are also part of the process of karma cleansing.

"No pain, no gain" may be a discredited maxim for athletic training, but it is a sacred spiritual law for the spiritual journey. Everyone on the spiritual journey will go through spiritual testing, which could take form as obstacles in any aspect of life. How does one overcome these obstacles and pass spiritual testing? The solution is to keep a clear mind and understand another spiritual law: "Success and disaster happen at the same time."

Do not worry about pain, and do not be afraid of disasters. Both are part of the process of purification, life transformation, and soul enlightenment. Do not let pain and disaster stop your growth. Be confident and patient as you take your spiritual journey. Trust in the Divine and in your spiritual guides. Offer unconditional love and service. With faith, trust, and love, soul enlightenment will come much faster.

Universal Meditation will offer great service for your spiritual journey. Practice it often as it will guide you step-by-step, further and further, helping you to fulfill your spiritual journey and to reach soul enlightenment. My message for all of you on the soul journey is: *I have the power to enlighten myself. You have the power to enlighten yourself. Together, we have the power to enlighten the world.*

Apply Universal Meditation to healing, blessing, harmonizing relationships, removing karma, transforming your life, and reaching soul enlightenment. Remember, anyone and everyone, anything and everything in the universe could be invited to join you, to bless you, and to offer service to one another — all inside your abdomen.

Be flexible and creative. All kinds of blessings can come to you from Universal Meditation. At the same time, practicing Universal Meditation allows you to offer service and blessings to the entire universe. This will only increase the blessings that you will receive.

Join me in a Universal Meditation to offer service to the entire universe to close this chapter:

> *Dear soul, mind, and body of the Divine, of all the Buddhas, saints, holy people, healing angels, archangels, ascended masters, enlightened teachers, and masters from every religion and belief system; dear soul, mind, and body of every city and country, of Mother Earth, of all the planets, galaxies, and universes; dear soul, mind, and body of everyone and everything in the universe, I love you. Could you all come into my abdomen?*
>
> *I am a universal servant. You are a universal servant. Everyone and everything is a universal servant. A universal servant offers universal service, including universal love, forgiveness, peace, healing, blessing, harmony, and enlightenment.*
>
> *Let us chant together to offer universal service unconditionally.*

Then chant the following ten mantras for one minute each:

> *Universal light, universal light, universal light, universal light.*
> *Universal servant, universal servant, universal servant, universal servant.*
> *Universal service, universal service, universal service, universal service.*
> *Universal love, universal love, universal love, universal love.*
> *Universal forgiveness, universal forgiveness, universal forgiveness, universal forgiveness.*

115

Universal peace, universal peace, universal peace, universal peace.

Universal healing, universal healing, universal healing, universal healing.

Universal blessing, universal blessing, universal blessing, universal blessing.

Universal harmony, universal harmony, universal harmony, universal harmony.

Universal enlightenment, universal enlightenment, universal enlightenment, universal enlightenment.

As you chant these mantras of universal service, visualize your abdomen holding the entire universe. Every soul of the universe is chanting with you. Every soul offers universal love, forgiveness, peace, healing, blessing, harmony, and enlightenment.

Close the meditation by thanking all the souls for their service, love, and blessings: *Thank you. Thank you. Thank you.* Then respectfully return them to where they came from: *Gong song. Gong song. Gong song.*

This is a truly *universal* meditation, because it gathers the energy of everyone and everything, of all souls in the universe. It is my great honor to lead you in this Universal Meditation to serve the entire universe.

Blessings. Blessings. Blessings.

Applications of Soul Mind Body Medicine

S oul Mind Body Medicine's addition of "soul over matter" to the "mind over matter" approach commonly taken by alternative medicines takes healing in a new direction. Practiced thousands of years ago, this ancient wisdom is only now being revealed.

This chapter focuses on practical healing applications of Soul Mind Body Medicine. Treat it as a healing encyclopedia for your health and wellness. In the first two sections, "The Four Power Techniques" and "Secret Energy Circles," I present more healing techniques. This material will give you an arsenal of powerful healing principles and methods to facilitate wellness of the physical, emotional, mental, and spiritual bodies. They are practical, easy to use, effective, and life transforming.

In the next sections of this chapter, I provide specific healing programs for losing weight, recovering from cancer, and healing emotional imbalances. The concluding sections reveal advanced wisdom about group healing, remote healing, and protection, and briefly introduce the concept of global healing. Then in chapter 7, "Using the Four Power Techniques to Heal Common Ailments," I offer a comprehensive guide for using the Four Power Techniques for the most common ailments that we all face.

Select the healing methods that most resonate with you and the healing programs that apply to you. Use them for your loved ones as well as for yourself. Remember, you have the power to heal yourself. Now go and do a good job!

THE FOUR POWER TECHNIQUES

The Four Power Techniques of Soul Mind Body Medicine can and should be used for almost all applications of this new medicine. Introduced in my previous book, *Power Healing*,[1] the techniques are Soul Power, Mind Power, Sound Power, and Body Power. Each technique practiced alone offers powerful healing, but it is much more powerful to use all four together. You have already been introduced to many applications of the Four Power Techniques in previous chapters of this book.

Why do we need to use all Four Power Techniques? Understand that an illness is much more than just a physical ailment. You must call on the power of the soul, mind, and body to heal on the physical, emotional, mental, and spiritual levels. Soul Power, Mind Power, Sound Power, and Body Power are simple yet powerful tools for doing this. As you practice the healing methods of Soul Mind Body Medicine, you will realize that although all four of these powers work together, the ultimate power is Soul Power. No healing can occur without the participation, agreement, and will of the soul. Soul Power is the underlying principle of Soul Mind Body Medicine and it is the reason why it is so effective. It cannot be emphasized enough: *Heal the soul first; then healing of the mind and body will follow.*

Let's briefly review the Four Power Techniques:

SOUL POWER. Soul Power is soul over matter, which means using the power of the soul to heal. The primary Soul Power technique in Soul Mind Body Medicine is Say Hello Healing (see chapter 2).

Say "hello" to the souls, and then request healing from them. We can say "hello" and request healing from the inner souls of our body, systems, organs, cells — even our DNA and RNA. We can also say "hello" to and request healing from the outer souls of nature, the universe, and the Divine.

SOUND POWER. Sound Power is the use of healing mantras and vibrational healing sounds. In chapter 4, I shared Weng Ar Hong, a powerful ancient healing mantra, along with some modern-day mantras.

MIND POWER. Mind Power is mind over matter, which means using the power of the mind, intention, creative visualization, and the potential of the brain to heal.

BODY POWER. Body Power refers to the use of specific hand positions for healing and for energy development. Especially significant is the One Hand Near, One Hand Far healing technique (see chapter 7) created by my master, Dr. Zhi Chen Guo. Various hand positions are used for healing different ailments. The positions work by creating energy fields of different densities. Energy flows naturally from a higher-density field of blocked energy to a lower-density field. Healing occurs when the energy blockage dissipates because energy can once again flow freely.

SECRET ENERGY CIRCLES

If, as the teaching has it, the human being is the small universe and all of nature is the big universe, then we must understand the small universe to understand the big universe, and vice versa. Whatever happens in the small universe also happens in the big universe, and the other way around.

Energy in the big universe generally flows through two main energy circles that circulate through the universe — the *horizontal energy circle* and the *vertical energy circle*. Replicating the universe, energy in the body also circulates through two main energy circles.

In the physical world, the horizontal and vertical energy circles represent the flow of energy in everything. For example, in mathematics, the x and y axes of the Cartesian plane represent horizontal and vertical energy circles. The Holy Cross is a similar representation, for in the spiritual world, the horizontal and vertical energy circles are the key circuits of energy flow for every soul of the universe. In the body, the horizontal energy circle is represented by the Dai meridian. The vertical energy circle is comprised of the Ren and Du meridians. Both are connected to the Chong meridian, which is also known as the Chong Mai, or Central meridian. These four major meridians of traditional Chinese medicine — the Ren, Du, Dai, and Chong — all have their starting point in the Snow Mountain Area energy center of the body (see figure 10).

Promoting energy flow in the horizontal and vertical energy circles

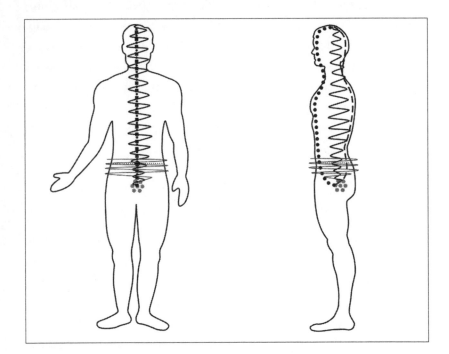

Figure 10. *The four major meridians start in the snow mountain area*

is critical for balancing one's soul, mind, and body. It is essential in achieving complete health on the physical, emotional, mental, and spiritual levels. Proper energy flow in these two primary energy circles prevents illness, maintains health, improves your quality of life, and prolongs life.

On a higher level, the horizontal and vertical energy circles are keys to transforming one's life and advancing enlightenment of the soul, mind, and body. On a universal level, these two energy circles bring world peace, harmony, and balance. In sum, proper flow of the horizontal and vertical energy circles is the key to harmony for both human beings and the universe.

Connect with the big universe when you promote energy flow in your horizontal and vertical energy circles. Request its blessings for your energy circles, and offer your service to the universe.

Practice with the Ren, Du, Dai, and Chong meridians to promote energy flow in your horizontal and vertical energy circles. The universe rejoices in the greater harmony that results. Enjoy the unlimited blessings of health and harmony that will come your way.

The Vertical Energy Circle

The vertical energy circle of the body is a loop of energy that circulates vertically through the Ren and Du meridians, commonly referred to as the Ren-Du meridians.

The Ren meridian starts from the Snow Mountain Area and flows up the *front* midline to the top of the head. It gathers the energy of six yin meridians: Liver, Heart, Spleen, Lung, Kidney, and Pericardium.

The Du meridian also starts from the Snow Mountain Area but flows up the *back* midline to the top of the head. It gathers the energy of six yang meridians: Gallbladder, Small Intestine, Stomach, Large Intestine, Bladder, and San Jiao (or the "three areas," referring to the Upper, Middle, and Lower Jiao. The Upper Jiao is the area of the body above the diaphragm. The Middle Jiao is the area between the diaphragm and the level of the navel. The Lower Jiao is the area from the navel down through the genitals. For good health, chi and bodily fluids must flow smoothly in the San Jiao).

The Ren and Du meridians connect to create the vertical energy circle. Thus combined, the Ren and Du meridians gather the energy of twelve other meridians. Promoting the energy flow of the Ren-Du meridians will promote energy flow of the ten major organs, the pericardium, and the San Jiao. This is a major but little-known method for healing all the major internal organs and the entire body.

How does one promote energy flow in this key energy circle of the body? We simply apply the Four Power Techniques:

BODY POWER. Sit on the floor in the full- or half-lotus position, or with your legs crossed naturally. You may also sit in a chair. Be comfortable, but keep your back straight, and do not lean back against the chair. Place the tip of your tongue close to, but not touching, the roof of your mouth. Contract your anus slightly. Close your eyes and relax.

To promote the vertical energy circle, you can use two different hand positions for Body Power. For either position, form a ring in each hand with your thumb and index finger. Keep the tips of those fingers close together, but not touching. Keep the other fingers curled and relaxed. Do this with both hands.

- *Flow in the Direction of Energy*: Hand Position A. Place both hands facing backward under each ear (see figure 11, p. 123). This hand position will make energy flow from the Snow Mountain Area, up the front midline along the Ren meridian to the top of the head, then down the back midline along the Du meridian back to the Snow Mountain Area. This is the direction of flow for energy in the body (see figure 12, p. 123).

- *Flow in the Direction of Matter*: Hand Position B. Hold both hands facing forward under each ear (see figure 13, p. 124). This hand position will make energy flow from the Snow Mountain Area up the back midline along the Du meridian to the top of

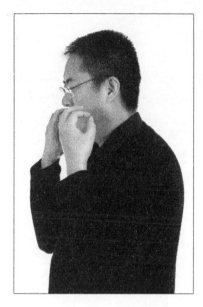

Figure 11.

Body Power (position A) for flow in the direction of energy

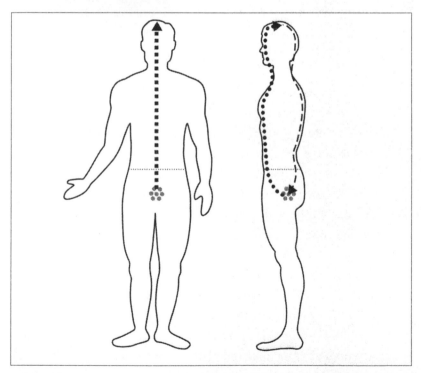

Figure 12. *Direction of energy flow*

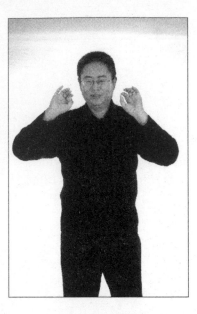

Figure 13.

*Body Power (position B) for
flow in the direction of matter*

the head, then down the front midline along the Ren meridian
back to the Snow Mountain Area. This is the direction of flow
for matter in the body (see figure 14, p. 125).

When you eat, matter (food) goes through the digestive tract,
through the esophagus to the stomach, then in turn to the small
and large intestines for absorption and storage, before being ex-
creted as waste through the anus. Hand Position B promotes this
flow of matter in the body.

When food goes through the digestive system, it stimulates
cellular vibration in the organs of the system (stomach, small and
large intestines), causing them to radiate energy into the space
between the organs. This energy flows up the front midline along
the Ren meridian to the top of the head, then flows down the back
midline along the Du meridian to the Snow Mountain Area. Hand
Position A promotes this energy flow in the body.

Hand Position B is the practice of most people, who are relatively limited to the material plane. Hand Position A is the practice of the saints, who are not limited in this way. Even though we
are human beings, we can practice the vertical energy circle using

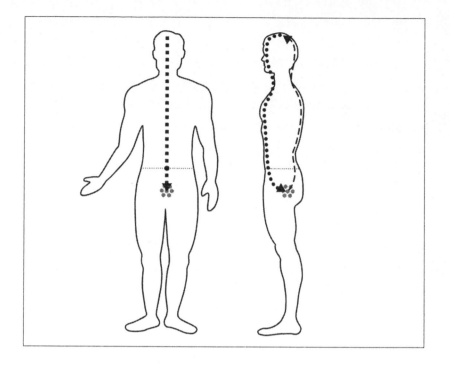

Figure 14. *Direction of matter flow*

both hand positions. Both are important and beneficial, but to develop your energy highly and to advance your spiritual journey toward the level of the saints, you must use Hand Position A.

SOUL POWER. Say "hello" to the meridians and ask them for healing: *Dear soul, mind, and body of my vertical energy circle, my Ren meridian, my Du meridian, the secret hand position,* dong, *the number zero* [see Sound Power below], *the golden light circle, I love you. Please promote energy and light flow in my Ren and Du meridians. Completely open my Ren-Du meridians. Clear all the blockages from my Ren-Du meridians to give me a total healing for my physical, emotional, mental, and spiritual bodies. You have the power to heal yourself. Please do a good job. Thank you. Thank you. Thank you.*

SOUND POWER. Chant the number zero in Chinese: *dong, dong, dong, dong* (pronounced "dōng"). Look at the numeral: o. It is rounded, an oval. It conveys the message of "circle," such an important meaning.

Now look around you. Look at the leaves on the trees. Most of them are round or oval. Have you ever seen a square leaf? Think about your cells, the smallest independently functioning unit of the body. They too are generally round or oval. So too are the cell organelles.

Energy flows in the body in a circle. Energy circles exist throughout the entire body, as well as within the organs, cells, DNA, and RNA. Energy flows through the universe in spirals, which are an infinite sequence of circles and ovals. These are the natural patterns of energy flow in the universe — always round, oval, or spiral. Energy doesn't flow in sharp angles, with abrupt changes of direction.

This simple and profound truth about the natural flow of energy in the universe is essential to understanding how to heal the soul, mind, and body. The knowledge that applies in the bigger universe also applies in the smaller universe of the human body. Use this wisdom when you heal yourself and others, in person or remotely. Rotate the healing light in round, oval, and spiral patterns. Apply this healing wisdom to people, animals, pets, flowers — anything at all.

MIND POWER. Visualize golden light flowing in a continuous vertical loop through the body along the Ren and Du meridians. The direction of flow will depend on which hand position you use.

When using Hand Position A, visualize a golden loop of light starting from the Snow Mountain Area flowing up the Ren meridian along the front midline to the top of the head, then flowing down the Du meridian along the back midline to the Snow Mountain Area. This saint's direction of the vertical energy circle promotes the flow of energy in the body.

When using Hand Position B, visualize a golden loop of light starting from the Snow Mountain Area flowing up the Du meridian along the back midline to the top of the head, then flowing down the Ren meridian along the front midline to the Snow Mountain Area. This normal person's direction of the vertical energy circle promotes the flow of matter in the body.

Summary: Practicing the Vertical Energy Circle

Practice the vertical energy circle by first positioning yourself comfortably. Select the hand position you are going to use. Activate your Soul Power by calling on the souls for healing. Then continuously chant *dong, dong, dong, dong*. At the same time, visualize the golden light circle looping around the vertical energy circle formed by the Ren-Du meridians. Visualize the light flowing faster and faster. Chant as fast as you can. Circulate the golden vertical circle as fast as you can.

Practice the vertical energy circle for *seven* minutes at a time. Observing the seven-minute practice rule is very important. Whether you practice once a day or many times per day, always practice for seven minutes.

This technique gives healing to all the major internal organs. Promoting flow in the vertical energy circle will improve the health of your physical, emotional, mental, and spiritual bodies immensely. You will get healing results beyond imagination.

The Horizontal Energy Circle

The horizontal energy circle of the body is a loop of energy that circulates horizontally through the body via the Dai meridian. Also referred to as the *belt* meridian, the Dai meridian is one of four major meridians starting from the Snow Mountain Area. From the front of the spinal column, the Dai meridian moves up to the level of the navel at the back before circulating inside the waist (see figure 15, p. 128).

In order to heal, maintain good health, and prevent illness, keep the energy flowing smoothly in this horizontal energy circle. Practice with the Dai meridian to open and develop its channel further.

The secret to opening your Dai meridian is to connect with the horizontal energy circles of the universe. Connect your small universe

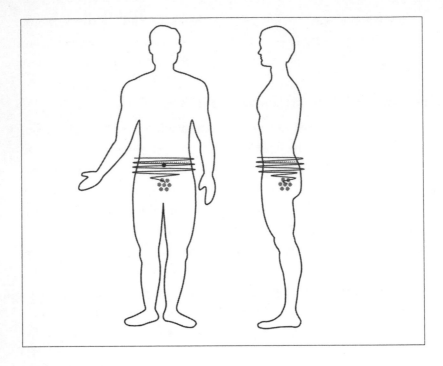

Figure 15. *The Dai meridian — horizontal energy circle*

with the big universe. When you practice with the horizontal energy circle (the Dai meridian), visualize your own horizontal energy circle connecting with the horizontal energy circles throughout the big universe. Connect with Mother Earth, every planet, every galaxy, and every universe. Connect with every tree, mountain, ocean, cloud, raindrop. Ask the souls, minds, and bodies of everyone and everything to practice with you to promote the flow of energy in their horizontal energy circles and to give a blessing for your horizontal energy circle.

Healing and blessings flow both ways. As you offer service to the entire universe, you receive blessings from the universe in return. Other souls appreciate your offering of service to them. The more you offer, the more blessings you will receive.

For healing applications, visualize the horizontal energy circle flowing continuously in your midsection. Golden light pours in from the universe and energizes the horizontal energy circle within your body. The horizontal energy circle can actually move up and down to any area of your body in need of healing. Make the golden light circle flow up to your head and down to your toes. Shrink and expand its circumference to move it inward from skin to bones and to any internal organ needing healing. Move the horizontal energy circle anywhere and everywhere to flow in every organ, every cell, every strand of DNA and RNA of your body. Apply the Four Power Techniques to promote horizontal energy flow in the Dai meridian:

BODY POWER. Sit on the floor in the full- or half-lotus position, or with your legs crossed naturally. You may also sit in a chair. Be comfortable, but keep your back straight, and do not lean back against the chair. Place the tip of your tongue close to, but not touching, the roof of your mouth. Contract your anus slightly. Close your eyes and relax.

Form a cage with your hands by pointing the fingertips of all five fingers closely at, but not touching, each other (see figure 16). Place your hands in this position in front of your abdomen without touching your body.

Your thumbs and index fingers will form a circle in front of your body. The secret of this hand position is that every finger represents the energy of a major internal organ, as summarized in table 3, p. 130. The thumb represents the energy of the spleen and stomach. The index finger represents the energy of the liver

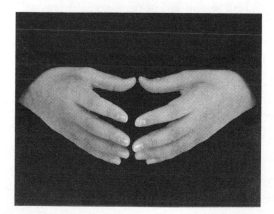

Figure 16.

Five Elements hand position for horizontal energy circle

and gallbladder. The middle finger represents the energy of the heart and small intestine. The ring finger represents the energy of the lungs and large intestine. The pinkie represents the energy of the kidneys and bladder. These organ pairs represent the Five Elements of traditional Chinese medicine: Wood, Fire, Earth, Metal, and Water.

Table 3. The Five Elements of the Fingers

Element	Yin Organ	Yang Organ	Finger
Wood	liver	gallbladder	index
Fire	heart	small intestine	middle
Earth	spleen	stomach	thumb
Metal	lungs	large intestine	ring
Water	kidneys	bladder	pinkie

The Body Power of this hand position promotes horizontal energy circle flow in all the organs of the Five Elements. Your hands literally form a horizontal energy circle. Each pair of fingers forms a horizontal energy circle with the thumbs. The fingers point at each other without touching for greater energy stimulation. Leaving a tiny gap between the fingers will stimulate much more cellular vibration in the fingers. All the organs of the Five Elements will receive the extra stimulus.

SOUL POWER. When you practice with the horizontal energy circle, ask the souls, minds, and bodies of the horizontal energy circle of Mother Earth, every planet, and every galaxy of the universe to practice along with you. Ask every one of them to join you in promoting the flow of their horizontal energy circles. At the same time, request the light of their horizontal energy circles to come to your own golden light circle. Here is an example of how to use Say Hello Healing when practicing the horizontal energy circle:

Dear soul, mind, and body of my Dai meridian;
Dear soul, mind, and body of my hand positions;
Dear soul, mind, and body of dong, *the number ʒero;*
Dear soul, mind, and body of my horiʒontal golden light circle;
Dear soul, mind, and body of the horiʒontal golden light circles of
*   Mother Earth, every planet, and every galaxy in the universe,*
I love you all. Please join with me.
You have incredible power to promote energy flow in my horiʒon-
*   tal energy circle and in everyone else's horiʒontal energy circle.*
*   Please give a blessing to everyone's horiʒontal energy circle,*
*   and bless my horiʒontal circle too.*
I am very honored and blessed. Thank you. Thank you. Thank you.

SOUND POWER. Chant the number zero in Chinese: *dong, dong, dong,*
dong. Chanting *dong* is a very special method for promoting energy flow in the proper circular, oval, and spiral patterns.

MIND POWER. Visualize a golden circle of light rotating around your
waist along the Dai meridian. You can visualize the light rotating
slowly or quickly, in larger or smaller circles, from skin to bone
in any part of your body. Rotate the golden light clockwise or
counterclockwise:

- *Clockwise*: Rotating the golden light circle clockwise is the
  horizontal energy circle practice of ordinary people. It is very
  important to rotate this circle as frequently and as quickly as
  you can.

- *Counterclockwise*: Rotating the golden light circle counterclockwise is the horizontal energy circle practice of the
  saints. If you want to develop your energy and advance your
  spiritual journey, clockwise practice is not enough; you must
  also practice rotating the horizontal energy circle counterclockwise.

Summary: Practicing the Horizontal Energy Circle

Place your hands in the Five Elements fingertip position near your abdomen (see figure 16, p. 129). Invoke Soul Power by saying "hello" to the inner and outer souls. Start chanting: *dong, dong, dong, dong.* Continue chanting throughout the practice. At the same time, visualize horizontal circles of golden light flowing and rotating in every system, organ, and cell of your body.

Visualize horizontal energy circles also circulating in every planet, every galaxy, and everything in the universe. Visualize one big horizontal energy circle of golden light flowing through the whole universe. Make the golden light circle of the universe flow faster and glow brighter. In this way, you are promoting horizontal energy circle flow for the entire universe.

Now place the horizontal energy circle of the universe in your body. The golden light of the universe merges with the light of your own horizontal energy circles. You are now practicing the Dai meridian with the horizontal energy circle of the whole universe flowing in your body and nourishing you. You are receiving healing for every system, organ, and cell of your body, right down to your DNA and RNA. The energy of the universe sends healing blessings to your physical, emotional, mental, and spiritual bodies.

Practice the horizontal energy circle energy flow for seven minutes at a time. Practice at least twice a day, the more often, the better. The healing blessings and spiritual nourishment you receive will be beyond measure.

The Chong Meridian

The Chong meridian is another of the four major meridians starting from the Snow Mountain Area. The Chong starts from the base of the spinal column, spirals up the front of the spinal column to the brain, and ends at top of the head (see figure 17, p. 133).

Recall that the Ren meridian gathers the energy of six yin meridians, and the Du meridian gathers the energy of six yang meridians. The energy gathered by these two meridians merges in the Chong meridian, or the Chong Mai, which translates as the "Central meridian."

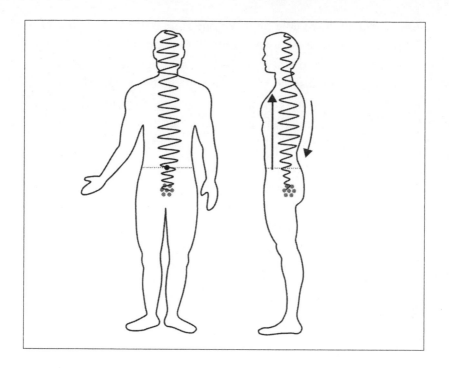

Figure 17. *The Chong meridian*

Consequently, the Chong meridian gathers the energy of fourteen meridians: the six yin meridians (Liver, Heart, Spleen, Lung, Kidney, Pericardium), the six yang meridians (Gallbladder, Small Intestine, Stomach, Large Intestine, Bladder, San Jiao), plus the Ren and Du meridians. Developing the Chong meridian promotes energy flow in fourteen meridians. Removing energy blockages in the Chong meridian is one of the most profound healing techniques.

You can develop the Chong meridian and remove energy blockages there by applying the Four Power Techniques:

BODY POWER. Sit on the floor in the full- or half-lotus position, or with your legs crossed naturally. You may also sit in a chair. Be comfortable, but keep your back straight, and do not lean back against the chair. Place the tip of your tongue close to, but not touching, the roof of your mouth. Contract your anus slightly. Close your eyes and relax.

Touch the middle finger of one hand to the top of your head at the Bai Hui acupuncture point. This point is located at the center of the top of the head at the intersection of a line drawn from the tip of the nose up to the back of the head and a line drawn from the top of one ear, up over the head, to the top of the other ear. Touch the middle finger of the other hand to your navel. Alternate hands if you get tired (see figure 18).

SOUL POWER. Say "hello" to the inner and outer souls and request a healing: *Dear soul, mind, and body of my Chong meridian; dear soul, mind, and body of my middle fingers; dear soul, mind, and body of Weng Ma Ni Ba Ma Hong* [see Sound Power below]; *dear soul, mind, and body of the golden light ball* [see Mind Power below], *I love you. You have the power to heal and develop my Chong meridian. Do a good job. Thank you. Thank you. Thank you.*

SOUND POWER. Weng Ma Ni Ba Ma Hong, pronounced "wung mah nee bah mah hōng," is the mantra of Guan Yin, the Goddess of Compassion, also known as Ling Hui Sheng Shi, which means "soul intelligence saint servant."

One of the most powerful healing and blessing mantras throughout history, Weng Ma Ni Ba Ma Hong has been chanted

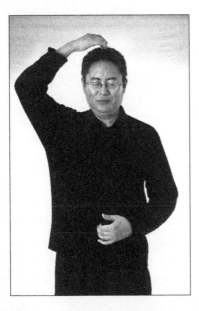

Figure 18.

Body Power for the Chong meridian

by millions of people. Chant this mantra to develop the power of the Chong meridian and to clear energy blockages from this channel. Chant *Weng Ma Ni Ba Ma Hong* for total healing of your physical, emotional, mental, and spiritual bodies.

MIND POWER. Visualize a golden light ball from the universe coming into the top of your head through the Bai Hui acupuncture point. This golden light ball is about two inches in diameter.

Rotating clockwise, it moves down the Chong meridian in front of your spine. After reaching the Snow Mountain Area, the golden light ball rotates counterclockwise back up the Chong meridian to the Bai Hui acupuncture point at the top of the head. In your visualization, repeat this down-and-up movement of the golden light ball.

Summary: Practicing with the Chong Meridian

Assume the Body Power position. Activate Soul Power by saying "hello" and requesting healing from the inner and outer souls. Chant *Weng Ma Ni Ba Ma Hong, Weng Ma Ni Ba Ma Hong, Weng Ma Ni Ba Ma Hong, Weng Ma Ni Ba Ma Hong* as quickly as you can throughout your practice.

At the same time, visualize a golden light ball from the universe entering the top of your head. Visualize it spiraling clockwise down the Chong meridian to the Snow Mountain Area. Then imagine it spiraling counterclockwise back up the Chong meridian to the top of the head. Visualize this golden light ball continuing to move up and down in this way.

Practice with the Chong meridian seven minutes per session, two or three times a day — the more, the better. Because promoting energy flow and removing energy blockages in the Chong meridian does the same in the Dai and Ren-Du meridians, Chong meridian practice is one of the most profound healing techniques you can learn. It promotes total healing of the physical, emotional, mental, and spiritual bodies by removing energy blockages from, and by developing, this channel. At the same time, you offer universal service during your practice. Chong meridian practice is simple, yet its healing results are beyond imagination.

Now we're ready for some specific healing programs using some of the Soul Mind Body Medicine techniques you have been introduced to.

WEIGHT LOSS

Soul Mind Body Medicine offers two very powerful exercises for those who want to lose some weight. The practice of the special mantras presented in chapter 4, Weng Ar Hong and 3396815, has been tailored to help you lose weight quickly and effectively. If you want to lose weight, practice these exercises using Soul Mind Body Medicine's Four Power Techniques at least twice a day for at least fifteen minutes at a time.

WENG AR HONG

You can combine the Four Power Techniques to support you in losing weight. Stand with your feet shoulder-width apart. Place your right hand a few inches above your navel and your left hand a few inches below the navel, with both palms facing up (see figure 8, p. 55). (If you have hypertension, headaches, a brain tumor, or brain cancer, turn the palm of your right hand to face downward.) When you are ready, ask the souls to help you lose weight: *Dear soul, mind, and body of every organ, every cell, I love you. Please increase your metabolism. Burn fat. You have the power to reduce my weight. Increase your metabolism. Do a good job. Thank you.*

Dear soul, mind, and body of Weng Ar Hong, I love you. You can stimulate the cellular vibration and increase the metabolism of every organ and cell of my body. Please do a good job. Thank you. Thank you. Thank you.

Then inhale deeply. As you exhale, chant: *W e e n n g g g,*

A a a a r r r r, H o o o n n g g in one long breath. Chant repeatedly. As you chant *Weng Ar Hong*, visualize bright red, bright white, and bright blue light, with each respective syllable, radiating in your head, chest, and abdomen. At the same time, visualize the bright light melting the fat in your body. Visualize yourself as slim and svelte. Continue chanting *Weng Ar Hong* and visualizing the light melting the fat in your body for at least fifteen minutes per session, twice a day, any time of the day.

3396815

Again, combine all Four Power Techniques. When you are properly seated, talk to your body: *Dear soul, mind, and body of my every organ and every cell, I love you. Please increase your metabolism. Burn fat. Adjust the functions of my endocrine system, digestive system, nervous system, circulatory system — all my systems — and balance my yin and yang to help me lose weight. Thank you.*

Dear soul, mind, and body of San San Jiu Liu Ba Yao Wu, *I love you. You can stimulate the cellular vibration and increase the metabolism of every organ and cell of my body. Please do a good job. Thank you. Thank you. Thank you.*

Then chant 3396815, *San San Jiu Liu Ba Yao Wu* as quickly as you can for fifteen minutes. At the same time, concentrate and visualize fire burning the fat from your organs, tissues, and cells. See your body becoming slimmer and slimmer. Keep these images in your mind's eye as you chant. Express your gratitude when you end the practice: *Thank you. Thank you. Thank you.* Practice at least twice a day.

These two techniques work so well because they combine Body Power, Soul Power, Sound Power, and Mind Power. These Four

Power Techniques stimulate the cellular vibration of every organ and cell in the body. Higher cell vibration increases the metabolic rate and adjusts the function of the systems, organs, and cells so that energy flows faster. Fat cells receive greater stimulus to release energy and revert to normal cells.

FOUR-WEEK RECOVERY PROGRAM FOR CANCER

Cancer, the great scourge of modern life, has become a dreaded disease in the West. Even after decades and billions of dollars of research, Western medicine has not found a cure. Nor does it understand the cause. Soul Mind Body Medicine sees cancer in a different light than most Western practitioners; it understands cancer to be the result of energy and spiritual blockages. More specifically, the emotional body of anger, which causes energy blockages in the liver, is probably the most common cause of all kinds of cancer.

Whether looking at the cause of illness from the viewpoint of Western medicine, traditional Chinese medicine, or any other healing modality, the common point is that illness affects cellular vibration. Western medicine does not give much attention to this concept but, as discussed in chapter 1, cellular vibration is a key to Soul Mind Body Medicine's understanding of the causes of all illnesses, including cancer. With this understanding, we can create an effective healing program for cancer.

The Matter Energy Message Theory (see chapter 1) explains how illness affects cellular vibration. To review, illness and cellular vibration can increase through any number of stimuli, including bacterial invasion, viral infection, trauma, injury, emotional imbalance, stress, genetic factors, and environmental conditions. When cells become overactive, they produce more energy. If energy cannot dissipate quickly enough from the area or organ, energy will accumulate in the space between the cells. As this concentration of energy builds, matter inside the cells is prevented from transforming to energy outside the cells.

Consequently, a blockage arises inside and outside the cells. Matter increases inside the cells, and energy increases outside the cells. Both matter and energy are prevented from undergoing their normal transformations of energy to matter and of matter to energy. Unresolved energy blockages result in illness and, over time, matter blockages cause normal cells to turn into precancerous cells, which can transform further into cancer cells if the matter blockages remain. Soul Mind Body Medicine therefore understands cancer as being caused by *too much matter inside the cells* and by *too much energy outside the cells*.

If energy and matter blockages cause cancer, the obvious solution would be to remove these blockages. Soul Mind Body Medicine begins cancer recovery by clearing the energy blockages. The secret to healing cancer is to *clean the space*, including the smaller spaces between the cells and the bigger spaces between the organs.

Energy blockages can also be caused by spiritual blockages, which arise from wrongdoing in lifetimes present and past. You carry this spiritual baggage as bad karma. To fully heal from cancer, you must not only clear the energy/matter blockages, but you must also clear the spiritual blockages. Recovery from cancer will be more effective if you follow the key principles of Soul Mind Body Medicine: heal the soul first; then healing of the mind and body will follow, and unconditional love, forgiveness, and service are the golden keys to healing.

In the following sections I will show you how to remove energy and spiritual blockages. These techniques have been successfully proven in China with thousands of cancer patients who have experienced marvelous healing results. When a documentary film producer went to China in 1999 to interview my teacher and master, Dr. Zhi Chen Guo, at his healing center, the producer asked how many in the audience of ten thousand had suffered from cancer. About two thousand cancer patients raised their hands. Then he asked how many had recovered and had experienced no recurrence of cancer for the last five years. More than half the cancer patients raised their hands. How did they achieve such an astounding success rate? They practiced Zhi

Neng Medicine, which is the foundation of Power Healing and Soul Mind Body Medicine. Since then, thousands more have successfully recovered from cancer by learning and practicing Zhi Neng Medicine.

These thousands of people in China and increasing numbers of people in the West have proven the efficacy of the cancer recovery program I am about to share with you. Although this cancer recovery program is based on Zhi Neng Medicine, it adds the powerful component of soul healing through Soul Power. The program can benefit anyone who has cancer, irrespective of type and stage at which it has been classified. Many cancer patients are fatigued and suffer terrible pain, depression, anger, sadness, and fear. Many others are confused and spiritually lost. This cancer recovery program will help you overcome many of these debilitating aspects of cancer, give you hope, ease your pain, and support your healing.

I offer these cancer recovery programs in support of all healing modalities. Use them to supplement and assist whatever cancer treatment you are also receiving. My intention is to let people know how they can assist their own cancer recovery by removing the energy and spiritual blockages in their lives. The wisdom and powerful healing tools presented here will assist cancer patients and healthcare practitioners everywhere.

Below I will outline an easy-to-follow and extremely effective four-week recovery program. The program consists of four practical exercises to be practiced daily. One by one, I will explain these powerful tools so you will understand how each one works and how to use them. In this four-week program, you practice the same four exercises every day at specific times. Your practice time increases each week, as summarized in table 4.

- Week 1: practice each exercise for at least five minutes a day.

- Week 2: practice each exercise for at least ten minutes a day.

- Week 3: practice each exercise for at least twenty minutes a day.

- Week 4: practice each exercise for at least thirty minutes a day.

After you have finished your first four weeks of practice, continue with the Week 4 practice schedule indefinitely until you are fully recovered. Keep in mind that cancer recovery may take months or years. Be patient and confident.

After you recover, continue practicing the Week 1 schedule, doing each of the four exercises for five minutes, for a total of twenty minutes of practice per day. Think of the Week 1 practice as preventive maintenance. It is important to maintain your good health, increasing your immunity and vitality, boosting your energy and stamina, and preventing reoccurrence. May you recover fully.

Table 4. Four-Week Cancer Recovery Program						
Continue with Week 4 practice until recovery. *Continue with Week 1 practice after recovery.*			Daily Practice (minutes)			
Practice Technique	When	Other Instructions	Week 1	Week 2	Week 3	Week 4
Weng Ar Hong	before breakfast	Face the sun and be with nature	5	10	20	30
Energy Booster	half hour after breakfast	Face the sun and be with nature	5	10	20	30
3396815	half hour after lunch	Face the sun (in the shade) and be with nature	5	10	20	30
Sha's Golden Healing Ball	half hour after dinner	Promote vertical and horizontal energy circles	5	10	20	30
Total daily practice time (minutes)			20	40	80	120

Cancer Recovery Practice One: Weng Ar Hong

Practice Weng Ar Hong (chapter 4, p. 54) diligently and sincerely as part of your daily morning routine. You will find that you have more energy and that your day will unfold with greater harmony.

- *When*: Early morning before breakfast.

- *Where*: The best setting in which to practice is outside facing the sun. If it is raining, cold, or you are too sick to go outside, then practice in your home. Try to open a window if you can, and face the sun. Facing the morning sun is important, since the sun carries tremendous healing power and nourishment for removing your energy and spiritual blockages. Practicing in natural surroundings is also very important for receiving the blessings of nature.

- *For How Long*: Practice daily for five minutes the first week, ten minutes the second week, twenty minutes the third week, and thirty minutes the fourth week. Practice longer for more healing.

- *How*: Apply the Four Power Techniques:

BODY POWER. Stand balanced and relaxed with your feet shoulder-width apart. Bend your knees slightly. If you are not able to stand, then sit or lie down. Keep your back straight. Place the tip of your tongue close to, but not touching, the roof of your mouth. Contract your anus slightly.

Hold your right hand, palm up, a few inches *above* the navel. Hold your left hand, palm up, a few inches *below* the navel (see figure 8, p. 55). Your hands should be close to, but not touching, your body to promote energy flow and healing. The same hand positions apply whether you are standing, sitting, or lying down, but it is best to practice Weng Ar Hong standing up. Note that your right hand should face palm *down* if you have hypertension, glaucoma, headaches, a brain tumor, or brain cancer.

SOUL POWER. Say "hello" to the inner and outer souls and ask them for healing: *Dear soul, mind, and body of all my systems, organs, cells, DNA, RNA, and the spaces between every cell and organ, I love you. You have the power to heal yourselves. Please do a good job. Thank you.*

Dear soul, mind, and body of the sun, please give me a blessing to heal me. You have the power to heal me. Do a good job. Thank you.

Dear soul, mind, and body of Weng Ar Hong, I love you. You have the power to heal me. Please do a good job. Thank you. I'm very honored and blessed. Thank you. Thank you. Thank you.

SOUND POWER AND MIND POWER. Take a deep breath after requesting healing blessings from the soul, mind, and body of all your systems, organs, cells, DNA, RNA, spaces, the sun, and Weng Ar Hong. As you exhale, chant *Weng Ar Hong* in one long breath. At the same time, visualize bright red light shining in your head when you chant *Weng*, bright white light shining in your chest when you chant *Ar*, and bright blue light shining in your abdomen when you chant *Hong*. Take another deep breath and repeat. Chant *Weng Ar Hong* repeatedly by sounding one repetition of it each time you exhale.

While you do this practice, think about and visualize being in perfect health. You *can* recover completely. Think about and visualize being healthy as often as possible, even when you are not practicing.

Weng Ar Hong and the San Jiao

As we know, in traditional Chinese Medicine, the San Jiao ("three areas") refers to the three main areas of the body and the organs and spaces within them. A large virtual organ, the San Jiao is the largest yang organ of the body.

The Upper Jiao is the area of the body above the diaphragm. It contains the heart, lungs, and brain. Its main functions are those of the heart and lungs, namely, blood circulation and respiration. The Middle Jiao is the area between the diaphragm and the navel. It contains the liver, gallbladder, stomach, pancreas, and spleen, and its main function is digestion. The Lower Jiao is the abdominal section below the navel and contains the bladder, the small and large intestines, the kidneys, and the reproductive organs. Its main functions are those of the kidneys, including water regulation. The San Jiao is summarized in table 5.

Table 5. The San Jiao			
San Jiao	Location	Organs	Main Functions
Upper Jiao	above the diaphragm	heart, lungs, brain	blood circulation, chi flow, and respiration
Middle Jiao	between the diaphragm and the navel	liver, stomach, gallbladder, pancreas, spleen	digestion
Lower Jiao	between the navel and the genital area	small and large intestines, urinary bladder, kidneys, adrenal glands, genitals, and reproductive organs	water balance and regulation

The San Jiao includes all the major organs of the body and serves as the passageway of chi and body fluids. Promoting the flow of chi and body fluids in the San Jiao removes energy blockages from the organs and the cells and promotes healthy organ functioning. Chanting *Weng Ar Hong* accomplishes this, because these sounds open the San Jiao by stimulating all its organs and cells. *Weng* stimulates cellular vibration in the brain. *Ar* stimulates cellular vibration in the entire chest, including the lungs and the heart. *Hong* stimulates cellular vibration in the entire abdomen, including the liver, stomach, gallbladder, spleen, small intestine, large intestine, kidneys, bladder, and reproductive organs.

Because Weng Ar Hong opens the San Jiao, it is very important for dissipating blocked energy (in the spaces). This in turn stimulates the clearing of matter blockages (inside the cells). Consequently, continued chanting of Weng Ar Hong can turn cancer cells, and precancerous cells, back into normal cells. Weng Ar Hong is a vital practice for healing, not only from cancer but from all illnesses.

Cancer Recovery Practice Two: Energy Booster

The Energy Booster technique will develop your stamina, increase your vitality, boost your immune system, and give you more energy. Practice consistently and diligently.

- *When*: A half hour after breakfast.

- *Where*: The best setting in which to practice is outside while facing the sun. If it is raining, cold, or you are too sick to go outside, then practice in your home. Whether indoors or out, always try to practice facing the sun.

- *For How Long*: Practice daily for five minutes the first week, ten minutes the second week, twenty minutes the third week, and thirty minutes the fourth week. Practice longer for more healing.

- *How*: Apply the Four Power Techniques:

BODY POWER. Sit in a chair or on the ground. Keep your back straight. If sitting in a chair, keep your feet flat on the floor. If sitting on the ground or on the floor, you can be in the lotus or half-lotus position (see figures 6 and 7, p. 53), or just cross your legs naturally. Place the tip of your tongue close to, but not touching, the roof of your mouth. Contract your anus slightly.

Hold your hands in the Yin/Yang Palm position (see figure 1, p. 43), with a firm grip. (Use about 80 percent of your full strength.) Place your Yin/Yang Palm against your lower abdomen.

SOUL POWER. Say "hello" to the inner and outer souls and ask them for healing: *Dear soul, mind, and body of my Lower Dan Tian, I love you. You are the foundational energy center of my body; key to immunity, stamina, vitality, and long life; and the seat of my soul. You are so important to my cancer recovery. Please do a good job building the power of my Lower Dan Tian. I am very honored and blessed.*

Dear soul, mind, and body of all planets, galaxies, and universes, including Mother Earth, could you send me your healing light from all directions? Pour through my skin into every part of my body to my Lower Dan Tian to form a light ball. I am honored and blessed. Thank you. Thank you. Thank you.

SOUND POWER AND MIND POWER. Repeatedly chant the number nine in Chinese, *jiu* (pronounced "joe"): *jiu, jiu, jiu, jiu....* Visualize the brightest golden, white, or rainbow light pouring in from the universe through every pore of your skin. The light penetrates your skin, muscles, tendons, organs, bones, and cells to focus in the Lower Dan Tian energy center. Concentrate more and more of this light from the universe in your Lower Dan Tian to form a solid golden light ball there. Visualize the universal light ball sending healing waves of love, nourishment, and compassion to all your cells.

The Energy Booster and the Lower Dan Tian

The Lower Dan Tian is the key energy center for immunity. The more you develop its power, the more energy, immunity, and life force you will have. Increasing your energy and revitalizing your immune system are extremely important in cancer recovery. By applying the Four Power Techniques in the Energy Booster exercise, you can spend five, ten, twenty, thirty minutes or more giving yourself an energy boost and building your Lower Dan Tian. You may feel hot, tingly, energized, and more alert after only five minutes of practice.

In the Mind Power visualization technique used in this exercise, the infinite light of the universe gives you incredible blessings. Entering through every pore of your skin, universal light washes through and nourishes all your organs and cells before concentrating in your

Lower Dan Tian to form a concentrated ball of light. Concentrate it more and more into a solid ball of light and universal life force. Feel it developing your Lower Dan Tian. Your abdomen may feel heavy and full.

This solid light ball has been part of many profound energy and spiritual practices for thousands of years. You can move the light ball to any part of your body for healing and blessing. Although not essential knowledge for this practice, be aware that the light ball can impart much more wisdom than healing and that its blessings are not restricted to the Lower Dan Tian. Blessings from the entire universe come to you in this simple yet powerful practice. Experience will make you a believer.

Practice the Energy Booster diligently, and it will boost your foundational power and increase your immunity, key in recovering from cancer.

Cancer Recovery Practice Three: 3396815

Ever since Dr. Zhi Chen Guo received the gift of 3396815 from the spiritual world, he has been teaching the use of this special number sequence as a secret mantra for healing and spiritual blessing. To review, 3396815, or *San San Jiu Liu Ba Yao Wu* in Chinese, is pronounced "sahn sahn joe lew bah yow woo." Many healing miracles and spiritual blessings have resulted from applying this secret mantra. Practice *San San Jiu Liu Ba Yao Wu* sincerely and consistently to restore your health.

- *When*: A half hour after lunch.

- *Where*: Practicing outside and facing the sun is best. If it is raining, cold, or you are too sick to go outside, then practice in your home. Whether indoors or outdoors, always try to practice facing the sun. Practice in the shade if the sun is too intense.

- *For How Long*: Practice daily for five minutes the first week, ten minutes the second week, twenty minutes the third week, and thirty minutes the fourth week. Practice longer for more healing.

- *How*: Apply the Four Power Techniques:

BODY POWER. Sit in a chair or on the ground. Keep your back straight. If sitting in a chair, keep your feet flat on the floor. If sitting on the ground, you can be in the lotus or half-lotus position, or just cross your legs naturally. Place the tip of your tongue close to, but not touching, the roof of your mouth. Contract your anus slightly.

Apply the One Hand Near, One Hand Far healing technique to your cancer. The Near Hand points to the area of cancer from four to seven inches away. Use whichever hand is most comfortable. If your arm tires, switch it to the Far Hand position and use the other hand as the Near Hand. If the cancer has metastasized, repeat the exercise with the Near Hand pointing at the other cancer areas. The Near Hand is the one that always points at the cancer.

Hold the Far Hand fifteen to twenty inches away from your body, with your palm facing your body. The Far Hand can face the lower abdomen, the lower back, or the side of your hip. If your cancer is in the lower abdomen, hold the Far Hand fifteen to twenty inches away facing your back. If you have cancer in the lower back, hold the Far Hand fifteen to twenty inches away facing the side of your hip.

SOUL POWER. Say "hello" to the inner and outer souls and ask them for healing: *Dear soul, mind, and body of my cancer cells, I love you. You have become abnormal. Please turn back into normal cells. You have the power to heal yourselves. Please do a good job. Thank you. Thank you. Thank you.*

Dear soul, mind, and body of 3396815, San San Jiu Liu Ba Yao Wu, I love you. You have the power to restore my health. Please give me a healing blessing. Thank you. Thank you. Thank you.

SOUND POWER. Chant the special healing mantra, 3396815, in Chinese, pronounced "sahn sahn joe lew bah yow woo."

MIND POWER. Chant *San San Jiu Liu Ba Yao Wu* repeatedly throughout the practice. At the same time, visualize bright light flowing continuously from the cancer area to the area facing the Far Hand. Usually this will be the Lower Dan Tian in your lower abdomen.

3396815, Energy Flow, and Healing

How does 3396815, *San San Jiu Liu Ba Yao Wu*, work? Why is this sequence of seven numbers so special and important in healing? To review, the sound of each number stimulates cellular vibration in a certain area of the body. *San san* (3, 3) stimulates cellular vibration in the lungs and chest, *jiu* (9) in the lower abdomen, *liu* (6) in the ribs, *ba* (8) in the navel, *yao* (1) in the head, and *wu* (5) in the stomach (see figure 19).

Chanting *3396815* causes energy to flow through the body in a specific and healthy pattern: chest → lower abdomen → both ribs → navel → head → stomach → chest, and so on. All the major internal organs

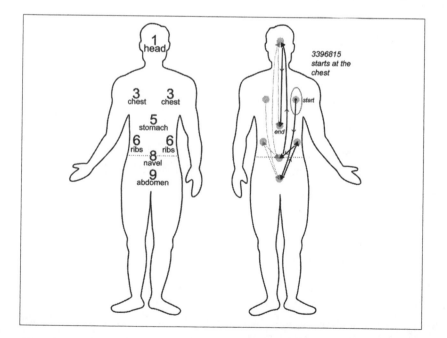

Figure 19. *3396815 and energy flow*

are appropriately stimulated in the right order. With continued practice, *San San Jiu Liu Ba Yao Wu* will balance and adjust your organs, remove energy and spiritual blockages, and open the spaces in your body.

Practice *San San Jiu Liu Ba Yao Wu* with dedication. The more you practice, the better. Healing happens every minute you chant this powerful mantra. By promoting a healthy and good flow of energy in your body, you will restore your health that much faster.

Cancer Recovery Practice Four: Sha's Golden Healing Ball

In chapter 4, I shared the story of how I received the divine gift of the Golden Healing Ball. Regardless of your belief system, this gift will serve anyone who requests and applies its healing blessings. Hundreds of thousands of people have used it to serve their healing and blessing needs. I am very honored and blessed to bring this gift to serve your soul, mind, and body in your recovery from cancer. Sincerely practice Sha's Golden Healing Ball to enhance your recovery.

- *When*: A half hour after dinner.

- *Where*: Practice indoors.

- *For How Long*: Practice daily for five minutes the first week, ten minutes the second week, twenty minutes the third week, and thirty minutes the fourth week. Practice longer for more healing.

- *How*: Apply the Four Power Techniques. This cancer recovery practice incorporates Sha's Golden Healing Ball in the practice of the vertical energy circle:

BODY POWER. Sit in a chair or on the ground. Keep your back straight. If sitting in a chair, keep your feet flat on the floor. In sitting on the ground, you can be in the lotus or half-lotus position, or just cross your legs naturally. Place the tip of your tongue close to, but not touching, the roof of your mouth. Contract your anus slightly.

Form an open ring in each hand with your thumb and index finger. Keep the tips of those fingers close together, but not touching. Keep the other fingers curled and relaxed. Do this with both hands. Place both hands facing *backward* under each ear (see figure 11, p. 123). This hand position promotes the vertical flow of energy in the body.

SOUL POWER. Say "hello" to the inner and outer souls and ask them for healing: *Dear soul, mind, and body of my vertical energy circle, I love you. You have the power to promote energy flow in yourself. Energy flow in your circle is one of the deepest secrets of healing. Please do a good job. Thank you. Thank you. Thank you.*

Dear soul, mind, and body of Sha's Golden Healing Ball, I love you. Please give me a healing blessing to promote energy flow in my vertical energy circle. I am honored and blessed. Thank you. Thank you. Thank you.

SOUND POWER AND MIND POWER. Chant the number zero in Chinese: *dong, dong, dong, dong.* Chant *dong* nonstop throughout the practice, as quickly as you can. Visualize Sha's Golden Healing Ball, starting from the Snow Mountain Area in front of the spine, flowing up the front midline to the top of the head, and then down the back midline to return to the Snow Mountain Area. Continue to visualize the ball looping around this vertical energy circle. The longer you can keep the vertical energy circle flowing, the more you will clear the blockages there to recover your health.

The vertical energy circle is a key energy circuit of the body. As long as energy is balanced and can flow smoothly through this circuit, all illnesses of the physical, emotional, and mental bodies can be healed.

This practice incorporates several important healing techniques. The hand position, the Body Power secret, promotes energy flow in the vertical energy circle. The Sound Power secret of *dong*, the number zero, also promotes energy flow in the vertical circle. The Mind Power secret is to visualize Sha's Golden Healing Ball flowing in the vertical energy circle. The Soul Power secret is to use Sha's Golden Healing Ball, a divine spiritual gift, to restore your health. As I've said many times, using all four secrets together is always much more powerful than applying the techniques individually.

⸙

You have now learned the four key practices of the Four-Week Cancer Recovery Program. As you chant the various mantras, try chanting out loud for about half the time and chanting silently for the remaining half of the time. Chanting aloud is yang chanting; it stimulates the larger cells of the body. Chanting silently is yin chanting; it stimulates the smaller cells. Alternating between chanting aloud and chanting silently alternates yang and yin healing of your cells. Giving yourself both kinds of healing is better than giving yourself only one kind.

Always give love to your cancer cells. Know that they can transform back into normal cells. Say "hello" to your cancer cells with the following message of Soul Power: *Dear soul, mind, and body of my cancer cells, I love you. You've gone in the wrong direction. Could you come back? Cancer cells, turn back to normal cells. You can do it. Do a good job. Thank you so much.* Remind your cancer cells that they are not in the right form. They will receive the message and begin to cooperate with you, if you only send them love.

Continue following the Cancer Recovery Program, following the week-by-week guidelines given above, indefinitely until you recover. Some people may recover in a matter of months, but for most, recovery from cancer can take a few years. Be patient. Be confident. Continue with other treatments you may be receiving, but keep practicing daily until you recover completely.

HEALING EMOTIONAL IMBALANCES

As we now know, human beings are composed of four interconnected bodies: the physical, the emotional, the mental, and the spiritual. Imbalance and illness in any one body will influence and can cause sickness in the other bodies.

The connection between the physical body and the emotional body was recognized thousands of years ago by Chinese medicine practitioners. From astute observations, ancient Chinese healers knew that liver illness in the physical body was linked with anger and rage in the emotional body. The converse was also true. They understood that unresolved anger in the emotional body could cause dysfunction of the liver, which could lead to other problems. In fact, Soul Mind Body Medicine considers anger to be the most common cause of cancer.

Similar links were observed between other emotions and the physical organs and are still valid today. People with heart problems are more prone to anxiety, depression, excitement, and joyful extremes in the emotional body. Conversely, long-term anxiety, depression, and too much excitement or happiness can give rise to heart problems. Spleen and stomach problems often result in worry, while worrying too much can generate spleen and stomach problems.

The interconnectedness of the emotional and the physical body extends to the emotions of grief and fear. If you have lung illness, you are more susceptible to sadness and grief, and vice versa. Kidney problems are connected with the emotional body of fear. For example, a common reaction to a sudden fright is the involuntary release of urine.

Before we proceed any further, you should know that traditional Chinese medicine and Western medicine have different concepts of the body's major internal organs. The Chinese understanding of an organ extends beyond and does not necessarily coincide with the anatomical and physiological functions understood by Western medicine.

The underlying concept is illness of the major organs in the physical body will cause unbalanced emotions in the emotional body, and vice versa. To heal the physical body one heals the emotional body, and vice versa. This was how Chinese medicine practitioners of old understood the relationship between the physical body and the emotional body. This relationship is summarized in table 6.

Table 6. Relationship between the Physical Body and the Emotional Body	
Physical Body Major Organ	Emotional Body Emotional Imbalance
liver and gallbladder	anger
heart and small intestine	depression, anxiety, overexcitement, too much joy
spleen and stomach	worry
lungs and large intestine	sadness, grief
kidneys and bladder	fear

Soul Mind Body Medicine recognizes interrelationships among all four bodies of existence. The physical, emotional, mental, and spiritual bodies are interconnected and interdependent. Illness and imbalance of one body will affect the health and balance of the other three.

Although the four bodies are interdependent, they are not equal in stature or importance. As we know, in Soul Mind Body Medicine, the controlling entity is the spiritual body. Nothing in your life can happen without the soul's consent, tacit or otherwise. The soul's dominance covers all matters, including life, death, love, finances — everything. This universal law gives rise to Soul Mind Body Medicine's guiding principle in healing. I will say it once again: *Heal the soul first; then healing of the mind and body will follow.*

The next few sections explain how to heal the emotional imbalances of anger, depression, anxiety, overexcitement, overjoy, worry, sadness, and fear using the Four Power Techniques. You will use Body Power, Soul Power, Sound Power, and Mind Power to heal the emotional body by removing energy blockages from the associated physical organs.

Anger

Anger is the emotional body connected with the liver. For example, people with a liver condition such as hepatitis, cirrhosis, or a tumor or cancer in the liver are generally easily upset. The converse is also true. If you are often angry and fly into rages at the slightest provocation, your constant anger hurts your liver by blocking its energy.

Think of the last time you argued so heatedly with your family or colleagues — or a stranger — that you lost your temper. Regardless of what upset you, you probably also lost your appetite at the time. Everybody has had this experience. When you are upset, anger stimulates the liver cells and makes them overactive. As a result, more energy than usual radiates from the liver, putting pressure on the stomach, which causes you to lose your appetite. Loss of appetite is only one of the first symptoms of liver stress caused by anger. Other manifestations can include poor digestion, liver disease, and cancer. Long-term anger like holding a perpetual grudge or flying into a rage all the time causes the liver to constantly radiate more energy. If the surrounding tissues and organs cannot dissipate this excess energy quickly enough, an energy blockage will build up in and around the liver. Over time, the blockage will result in liver dysfunction, liver disease, and other complications such as cancer.

To heal yourself and others of anger, the simple solution is to remove the energy blockage in the liver area.

Apply the Four Power Techniques to heal the unbalanced emotional body of anger:

BODY POWER. Use the One Hand Near, One Hand Far healing technique. Point the Near Hand at the liver, from four to seven inches away. Hold the Far Hand fifteen to twenty inches away from your body with the palm facing the lower abdomen, as shown in figure 20. The Near Hand creates a high-density field at the liver, while the Far Hand creates a low-density field at the lower abdomen. Energy will flow from the high-density field to the low-density field. In this case, energy will flow from the liver to the lower abdomen and dissipate the energy blockage in the liver.

SOUL POWER. Say "hello" to the soul of your liver and ask it for healing: *Dear soul, mind, and body of my liver, I love you. Your energy is blocked. You have the power to heal yourself. Do a good job. Thank you.*

Dear soul, mind, and body of chee [Chinese pronunciation of the number seven] *and joe* [Chinese pronunciation of the number nine], *I love you. You have the power to heal my anger. Do a good job. Thank you.*

SOUND POWER. Chant the number seven, pronounced "chee" in Chinese, and the number nine, pronounced "joe" in Chinese. *Chee* vibrates the cells of the liver. *Joe* vibrates the cells of the lower abdomen. Put them together and repeatedly chant *chee joe, chee joe, chee joe, chee joe.* Chanting *chee joe* helps transfer energy from the liver to the lower abdomen. Chant aloud or silently as quickly as you can. Also, chant *I love my liver, I love my liver, I love my liver, I love my liver* from time to time.

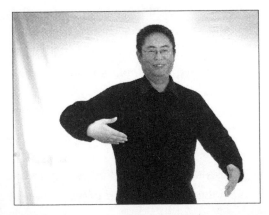

Figure 20.

Body Power for healing anger

MIND POWER. Visualize a stream of golden light flowing from the liver to the lower abdomen. The light continually transfers blocked energy from your liver to your lower abdomen. Visualize your liver itself glowing with bright green light and being free of obstructions. (According to the Five Elements theory of traditional Chinese medicine, green is the color associated with the Wood element and the liver.)

Practice for three to five minutes at a time, several times a day. Maintain the One Hand Near, One Hand Far Body Power position throughout the practice.

These powerful healing techniques will cause energy to flow from the liver to the lower abdomen. As you practice more, the energy you dissipate from the liver will further remove the energy blockage there. Continue this healing practice until your anger is healed. As you heal, you may notice other benefits, such as improvement in tendon and eye conditions, more energy, better digestion, a happier disposition, and even recovery from cancer. You *can* heal your anger and your liver.

Depression, Anxiety, Overexcitement, and Overjoy

Happiness is a major emotional factor affecting the heart. Although laughter is a wonderful healer, too much laughter and too much happiness are actually not good for the heart. In fact, too much happiness and excitation can cause a heart attack.

You may have friends or family members who became overly excited and subsequently suffered a heart attack. Why? The heart got so excited that its blood flow was blocked by the energy that accumulated. Overexcitement causes the heart to beat very quickly, sometimes too quickly for the amount of blood and oxygen it receives. A heart attack happens when the heart cannot supply enough blood to the body.

Other emotional factors linked to the heart include anxiety and depression. Everyone has been anxious or depressed at some point, but excessive anxiety can lead to paranoia, and deep depression can be debilitating and even cause you to be self-destructive. Both conditions can severely diminish one's quality of life.

In my many years of study and healing, I have come to an understanding of depression and anxiety that I would like to share with you. Depression and anxiety are energy blockages in the area of the heart and the Message Center. To review, the Message Center, or heart chakra, is a fist-sized energy center located behind the sternum in the middle of the chest. It is the spiritual communication center of the body. Its development allows you to communicate directly with the Divine and the souls of the universe on a spiritual basis. Blockages in the Message Center impede the development of your spiritual, mental, and emotional bodies.

The emotional extremes of overexcitement, overjoy, depression, and anxiety are all blockages in the Message Center. Heal these unbalanced emotions by removing the energy and spiritual blockages from the Message Center.

Apply the Four Power Techniques to heal emotional imbalances of the heart:

BODY POWER. Use the One Hand Near, One Hand Far healing technique. Point the Near Hand at the center of the chest, from four to seven inches away. Hold the Far Hand fifteen to twenty inches away from your body with the palm facing the lower abdomen, as shown in figure 21. The Near Hand creates a high-density field at the Message Center, while the Far Hand creates a low-density field at the lower abdomen. Energy will flow from the high-density field to the low-density field. In this case, energy will flow from the Message Center to the lower abdomen and dissipate the energy blockage in the Message Center.

SOUL POWER. Say "hello" to the souls of your Message Center and others and ask them for healing: *Dear soul, mind, and body of my Message Center, my lower abdomen, my near hand and far hand,* sahn, *and* joe, *I love you all. You have the power to heal my depression, anxiety, overexcitement, and/or overjoy. Do a good job. Thank you.*

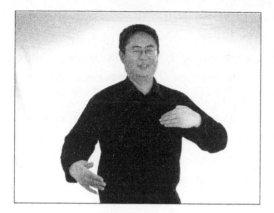

Figure 21.

Body Power for healing depression and anxiety

The Soul Power of all these souls will actively join together to heal the emotional body of your Message Center.

SOUND POWER. Chant the number three, pronounced "sahn" in Chinese, and the number nine, pronounced "joe" in Chinese. *Sahn* vibrates the cells of the Message Center. *Joe* vibrates the cells of the lower abdomen. Put them together and repeatedly chant *sahn joe, sahn joe, sahn joe, sahn joe.* Chanting *sahn joe* helps transfer energy from the Message Center to the lower abdomen. Chant aloud or silently as quickly as you can. Also, chant *open Message Center, open Message Center, open Message Center, open Message Center* from time to time.

MIND POWER. Visualize the brightest golden light flowing from the Message Center to the lower abdomen. The light continually transfers blocked energy from your Message Center to your lower abdomen. Visualize your Message Center being clear of obstructions.

Practice for three to five minutes at a time, several times a day. Maintain the One Hand Near, One Hand Far Body Power position throughout the practice. You *can* heal your depression, anxiety, overexcitement, overjoy, and your heart.

Worry

In traditional Chinese medicine, the spleen is the major organ responsible for digestion. It is also responsible for controlling blood flow and keeping blood in the vessels. It is connected with the muscles, mouth, and lips, and with the emotional body of worry. Consequently, any dysfunction of the spleen can result in worry, muscle problems, sores or cankers in the mouth, and swollen lips. The converse is also true; any of these conditions can cause blockage in the spleen.

Worrying is a natural aspect of being human. However, when we worry too much, we need to address this problem by understanding that worry is the emotional body connected with the spleen. The solution for worry in Soul Mind Body Medicine is to remove the energy blockage there.

Apply the Four Power Techniques to heal the unbalanced emotional body of worry:

BODY POWER. Use the One Hand Near, One Hand Far healing technique. Point the Near Hand at the spleen, from four to seven inches away. The spleen is located just under the diaphragm inside the left rib cage. Hold the Far Hand fifteen to twenty inches away from your body with the palm facing the lower abdomen, as shown in figure 22. The Near Hand creates a high-density field at the spleen, while the Far Hand creates a low-density field at the lower abdomen. Energy will flow from the high-density field to the low-density field. In this case, energy will flow from the spleen to the lower abdomen and dissipate the energy blockage in the spleen.

SOUL POWER. Say "hello" to the soul of your spleen and ask it for healing: *Dear soul, mind, and body of my spleen, I love you. Your energy is blocked. You have the power to heal yourself. Do a good job. Thank you.*

Dear soul, mind, and body of woo [Chinese pronunciation of the number five] *and* joe [Chinese pronunciation of the number nine], *of my near hand and far hand, of my lower abdomen, and of the brightest golden light, I love you. You have the power to heal my worry. Do a good job. Thank you.*

SOUND POWER. Chant the number five, pronounced "woo" in Chinese, and the number nine, pronounced "joe" in Chinese. *Woo*

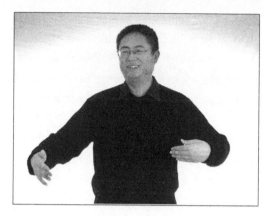

Figure 22.

Body Power for healing worry

vibrates the cells of the spleen. *Joe* vibrates the cells of the lower abdomen. Put them together and repeatedly chant woo joe, woo joe, woo joe, woo joe. Chanting *woo joe* helps transfer energy from the spleen to the lower abdomen. Chant aloud or silently as quickly as you can. Also, chant *I love my spleen, I love my spleen, I love my spleen, I love my spleen from time to time.*

MIND POWER. Visualize a stream of bright golden light flowing from the spleen to the lower abdomen. The light continually transfers blocked energy from your spleen to your lower abdomen. Visualize your spleen itself as happy, healthy, and free of blockages.

Practice for three to five minutes at a time, several times a day. Maintain the One Hand Near, One Hand Far Body Power position throughout the practice. You *can* heal your worry and your spleen.

Grief and Sadness

Westerners think of the lungs primarily as a respiratory organ. In traditional Chinese medicine, the lungs are connected with body chi and respiratory chi, and the nose. The lungs also assist in water metabolism and are associated with the emotions of grief and sadness. (Think of a sigh.) Those who follow Eastern spiritual practices know the lungs to be the part of the body that belongs to Heaven.

Soul Mind Body Medicine considers grief and sadness to be energy blockage in the lungs. Losing someone you love can make you so sad that your lungs become blocked. When the lungs are blocked, it is easy to catch cold, tire quickly, and be even more susceptible to sadness. The healing solution for grief and sadness is to remove the energy blockage in the lungs. Simply apply the Four Power Techniques:

BODY POWER. Use the One Hand Near, One Hand Far healing technique. Point the Near Hand at your lungs, from four to seven inches away. Hold the Far Hand fifteen to twenty inches away from your body, with the palm facing the lower abdomen as in figure 23. The Near Hand creates a high-density field at the lungs, while the Far Hand creates a low-density field at the lower abdomen. Energy will flow from the lungs to the lower abdomen, dissipating the energy blockage in the lungs.

SOUL POWER. Say "hello" to the soul of your lungs and the other souls and ask them for healing: *Dear soul, mind, and body of my lungs, my lower abdomen, my near hand and far hand, sahn, and joe, and the brightest golden light, I love you. You have the power to heal my grief and sadness. Do a good job. Thank you.*

SOUND POWER. Chant the number three, pronounced "sahn" in Chinese, and the number nine, pronounced "joe" in Chinese. *Sahn* vibrates the cells of the lungs and chest. *Joe* vibrates the cells of the lower abdomen. Put them together and repeatedly chant *sahn joe, sahn joe, sahn joe, sahn joe*. Chanting *sahn joe* helps transfer energy from the lungs to the lower abdomen. Chant aloud or silently as quickly as you can.

MIND POWER. Visualize the brightest golden light flowing from the lungs to the lower abdomen. Use the intention of your mind and the power of creative visualization to transfer blocked energy from your lungs to your lower abdomen.

Practice for three to five minutes at a time, several times a day. Maintain the One Hand Near, One Hand Far Body Power position throughout the practice. You *can* heal your grief, your sadness, and your lungs.

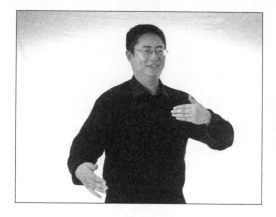

Figure 23.

Body Power for healing grief and sadness

Fear

The emotional body of fear is connected with the kidneys. When you are frightened, fear weakens your kidneys. Conversely, if your kidneys are weak, you tend to frighten more easily and, in the extreme, to be paranoid. The healing solution for fear is to remove the energy blockage in the kidneys. Use the Four Power Techniques:

BODY POWER. Use the One Hand Near, One Hand Far healing technique. Hold the Near Hand four to seven inches behind your back with the palm facing one of the kidneys. The kidneys are located on either side of your back two or three inches above waist level. Hold the Far Hand fifteen to twenty inches away from the body with the palm facing the ribs on the opposite side (see figure 24, p. 164. The Near Hand creates a high-density field in the area of the kidney. The Far Hand creates a low-density field in the area of the ribs. Energy will flow from the kidneys to the area of the ribs. If you get tired, alternate your hands to face the other kidney and the ribs on the other side.

SOUL POWER. Say "hello" to the soul of your kidneys and the other souls and ask them for healing: *Dear soul, mind, and body of my kidneys, my ribs, my near hand and far hand,* joe [Chinese pronunciation of the number nine] *and* lew [Chinese pronunciation of the number six], *and the brightest golden light, I love you all. You have the power to heal my fear. Do a good job. Thank you.*

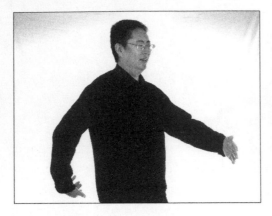

Figure 24.

Body Power for healing fear

The Soul Power of all these souls will actively join together to heal your fear.

SOUND POWER. Chant the number nine, pronounced "joe" in Chinese, and the number six, pronounced "lew" in Chinese. *Joe* vibrates the cells of the lower abdomen, including the kidneys. *Lew* vibrates the cells of the rib area. Put them together and repeatedly chant *joe lew, joe lew, joe lew, joe lew*. Chanting *joe lew* helps transfer energy from the kidneys to the rib area. Chant aloud or silently as quickly as you can.

MIND POWER. Visualize the brightest golden light flowing from the kidneys to the rib area. Mind Power helps to remove the energy blockage in the kidneys and to heal your fear.

Practice for three to five minutes at a time, several times a day. Maintain the One Hand Near, One Hand Far Body Power position throughout the practice. You *can* heal your fear and your kidneys.

BROADER APPLICATIONS OF SOUL MIND BODY MEDICINE

So far in this chapter we have discussed some very specific applications of Soul Mind Body Medicine, but its applications are much broader. Can you use Soul Mind Body Medicine to offer healing to a group of people? Can you use it to offer healing to someone on the other side of the planet? Can it help protect you from people who stress you out and drain your energy? Can it help heal Mother Earth? The answer to all these questions is yes! Below we will explore how.

Group Healing

Imagine you have a group of twenty, two hundred, two thousand, twenty thousand, or even 2 million people in front of you. Everyone in the group has his or her own specific health concerns or illnesses. You can offer healing to everyone in the group at the same time through the practice of what I call group healing.

In China, I have had many experiences of offering group healing to gatherings of more than ten thousand people at once. Below I will share some of the techniques you can use. The most important thing to remember is: *I can do it. You can do it. I have the power to heal myself. You have the power to heal yourself. Together, we have the power to heal the world.*

Group healing works, no matter what kinds of illnesses or health problems those in the group have. It is equally effective applied to a group of people with the same health condition (for example, arthritis) or to a group of people with diverse health concerns. You do not need to think about healing the specific illnesses or concerns of the group. You do not even need to know what any of these illnesses or concerns are!

When you offer group healing, you can ask everyone to identify and make his or her own healing request. They may make their requests aloud or silently, privately or publicly. After everyone has made a healing request, you can offer group healing to address all the healing requests the group has made. It takes only a few minutes. Use the Four Power Techniques together to offer group healing:

SOUL POWER. Start by making a sincere request to the soul world. Say "hello" to the souls of everyone that you will offer healing to, and ask them to heal themselves. Say "hello" to the holy beings and ask for their help in healing. Ask the souls of nature and of the universe for their healing blessings as well. Here is an example of how to invoke soul healing on behalf of the group. You can be creative in customizing and personalizing it: *Dear soul, mind, and body of everyone in the group, I love you. You can use your own Soul Power and Mind Power to help yourself. Do a good job. The power of my soul, mind, and body is at your service. I offer my healing to you.*

Dear soul, mind, and body of all the healing angels, Buddhas, saints, gurus, spiritual guides, and teachers, we love you. You have incredible healing power. Please bless this group to heal their physical, emotional, mental, and spiritual bodies.

Dear soul, mind, and body of Mother Earth, all the oceans, mountains, rivers, trees, flowers, cities, and countries, we love you. Could you come here to give a healing blessing to this group?

Dear soul, mind, and body of the sun, moon, all the planets, all the stars, all the galaxies, and all the universes, we love you. Could you give a healing blessing to this group to heal their souls, minds, and bodies?

Dear soul, mind, and body of universal light, we love you. You have the power to heal everyone. Could you come to this group and wash through everyone, from head to toe, from skin to bone, to all the cells? Please give a healing blessing to remove blockages at the cellular level for everyone's souls, minds, and bodies.

We ask for total healing of the physical, emotional, mental, and spiritual bodies. We are deeply honored and blessed. Thank you. Thank you. Thank you.

BODY POWER. Extend one hand to point at the group (see figure 25, p. 167). Alternatively, hold out both hands to enfold and embrace the group in the healing blessings you call forth. Hold either hand position for the duration of the healing.

SOUND POWER. Chant continuously: *universal light, universal light, universal light, universal light.*

MIND POWER. Visualize the brightest golden, purple, or rainbow light of the universe washing through everyone in the group, from

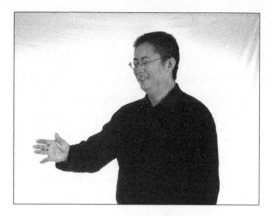

Figure 25.

One-Hand Healing technique

head to toe, skin to bone. This universal light penetrates every-one's cells, removing blockages at the cellular level. Healing hap-pens as everyone is bathed in the healing light of the universe.

After three to five minutes, end the group healing by thank-ing all the souls for their healing blessings: *Thank you. Thank you. Thank you.* Then respectfully return the souls who came: *Gong song. Gong song. Gong song.*

This technique reveals the simple yet profound secrets of group healing. The practice incorporates a very deep and power-ful truth recognized long ago: *The universe is one. The Divine is one.*

All are one. By healing one, you heal all.

Remote Healing

Quantum physicists of the twentieth century concluded that *there is no space or time*. Spiritual practitioners knew and practiced this con-cept thousands of years ago. The Universal Meditations of Soul Mind Body Medicine are an example of Lao Tzu's statement "Stay at home to know the universe." The universe is in every cell of your body, in a tree, in a flower, even in a grain of sand. And, as we learned in the last chapter, the Buddhists teach, "One grain of sand holds three thousand universes," meaning the tiniest thing in the universe holds the entire universe. This deep spiritual wisdom also applies to healing.

You may be in North America while the person you are concerned about is in Europe. You could be in China and learn that your brother in South Africa is ill. You could be at work worried about your father, who has just suffered a stroke and is lying paralyzed in the local hospital. You can help them with remote healing.

By definition, remote healing is not dependent on physical proximity. It doesn't matter how near or how far you are from the object of your healing. Just think of the person you are sending healing to, and their soul will be immediately before you. Whatever healing you can offer to anyone physically in front of you, you can also do remotely. Essentially, remote healing is no different from healing in person. The speed of thought, message, and healing is faster than the speed of light.

Let's say you want to offer remote healing to your sister, who is halfway around the world and suffering from shoulder pain. You can phone her and give her remote healing while you are connected by phone. Alternatively, you can give her remote healing without even being together on the phone. In the first instance, your sister is aware that you are giving her healing; in the second, she is not. Both ways are equally effective.

Sometimes remote healing can be better and more powerful than in-person healing. However, most people prefer the personal touch, since that is what they are used to. The energy from remote healing can be very strong, so it is most effective when the recipient can close his or her eyes and relax, even sleep. As the healer, if you have a few minutes in the evening or upon awakening, you could offer a remote healing in one or two minutes. Miracles can happen for the recipients.

All the healing techniques introduced in this book can be used for remote healing. Even though the healing recipient is not physically in your presence, you can call the recipient's spiritual presence to come before you. For example, you could ask the soul of your sister: *Could you come and stand in front of me?* You could also call her soul to lie down in front of you as you offer the healing, or you can simply think about your sister, wherever she may be. She may be asleep, she may be working, she may be traveling — it doesn't matter. As long as you call your sister's soul or think about her, her soul (actually, her *subdivided* soul) will be in front of you.

Once you have summoned the soul of your sister, apply the Four Power Techniques to offer her healing. You could point your hand at her soul, chant healing number sounds and mantras, visualize bright light flowing through her soul to remove blockages and apply Say Hello Healing, as described below. As with all techniques of Soul Mind Body Medicine, you are applying healing on the level of the soul. Your sister's mind, emotions, and body will receive healing at the same time. Soul Healing naturally translates to physical, emotional, and mental healing because the soul, mind, and body are closely connected, and the soul is always the boss.

Say "Hello"

Invoke the power of the soul to heal itself: *Dear soul, mind, and body of my sister, I love you. Dear soul, mind, and body of my sister's shoulder* [for example], *I love you. You have the power to heal yourselves. Please do a good job. I am also going to send a healing to you.* The simple act of saying "hello" to your sister's soul initiates a healing reaction in her body. This Soul Healing component is absolutely key to remote healing.

Next, say "hello" to the healing mantras or souls of nature and ask them to support your remote healing by adding their healing blessings. For example: *Dear soul, mind, and body of* San San Jiu Liu Ba Yao Wu (3396815), *I love you. Can you offer a healing blessing to my sister's shoulder?* Then chant *San San Jiu Liu Ba Yao Wu.* Or, *Dear soul, mind, and body of Weng Ar Hong, could you offer healing to my sister?* Then chant *Weng Ar Hong.*

Pointing with One Hand

Extend one hand and point to the soul of your sister, which you have called before you (see figure 25, p. 167). Visualize your sister's image in front of you. This is the Body Power component of remote healing. This One-Hand Healing technique reinforces the connection between you and your sister's soul.

Sound Power

Chant the mantras or the healing number sounds you have requested when you said "hello." Chant for at least one minute, aloud or silently.

Visualization

Visualize bright golden light in your sister's shoulder. Or, you could request and visualize Sha's Golden Healing Ball spinning in your sister's shoulder or simply bright golden light flowing in your sister from head to toe. Another option is to apply the technique of Universal Meditation by visualizing your sister inside your abdomen and enveloping her and her shoulder in the love and light of the universe.

Duration of Healing

You can offer remote healing for as little as one minute, using the One-Minute Healing method. Alternatively, you can practice remote healing for three to five minutes, as will be specified in chapter 7, "Using the Four Power Techniques to Heal Common Ailments." Of course, you can offer remote healing for as long as you wish.

Perhaps you will be able to remove the energy blockage in your sister's shoulder just by offering remote healing once. In any case, continue to offer remote healing as long as her condition lasts. One day, your sister will find the pain in her shoulder dissipating and her shoulder healing.

Give Thanks

In practicing remote healing and all the methods of Soul Mind Body Medicine, gratitude is a very necessary and serious spiritual requirement. You can ask the souls of the saints, Buddhas, healing angels, the sun, moon, stars, and so on for their healing blessings, but you must remember to appreciate them sincerely and to thank them. Do not forget to honor them for their responsiveness to your request for blessings and healing. Conclude your remote healing session by saying: *Thank you, thank you, thank you. Gong song, gong song, gong song.*

Protection

Have you ever noticed how other people's energy can sometimes be detrimental to you? For example, you find yourself emulating a friend's bad behavior, or you seem to be more critical after spending time with someone who often puts other people down. You might also notice that you feel drained every time your perpetually down-on-her-luck friend phones you. Or that you have to be careful about being around people you don't like, otherwise you get sad or angry, risking an instant asthma attack. Or you wonder why contact with a certain person seems to bring out your worst qualities. Sometimes, you won't even leave home so as to avoid meeting certain people.

All these situations can affect the quality of your life physically, emotionally, mentally, and spiritually. In some cases, they can be extremely debilitating and damaging if they affect your health and the safety of your loved ones. How can you protect yourself so that other people's energy doesn't interfere with you or make you unhealthy?

Soul Mind Body Medicine offers several powerful techniques for protecting yourself before you go out in public or before meeting people you don't like. Simply apply Say Hello Healing and ask for protection from a powerful mantra, holy being, or spiritual healing tool such as *San San Jiu Liu Ba Yao Wu*, Guan Yin, Jesus, or Sha's Golden Healing Ball: *Dear soul, mind, and body of Sha's Golden Healing Ball, I love you. Can you totally cover and protect me inside and out for the whole day? For the next twelve hours, help me to stay calm. Continue to rotate all around me and within me. I am so honored. Thank you.* Sha's Golden Healing Ball will instantly surround and shield you inside and out, giving you the protection you requested.

You could chant *San San Jiu Liu Ba Yao Wu* or *universal light* silently. You could ask for protection from Mother Mary, Shiva, Guan Yin, or God. Select one mantra or highest being, and ask it to protect you. Your energy field will be protected by the Divine. You will find that you are not as easily upset or as emotional as usual, and that other people's energy hardly affects you anymore. If you do encounter unpleasant energy, it cannot attack you because of the strength of your divine protection field.

You can use the same technique to protect others. You may be worried about your young child going off to school on his own. Give him protection in the same way before he leaves home. Apply Say Hello Healing and invoke the protection of a favored saint, Buddha, or mantra. For example, you could ask Lao Tzu to protect your child: *Dear Lao Tzu, I love you. Could you protect my child?* You could also ask Sha's Golden Healing Ball for protection: *Dear Sha's Golden Healing Ball, can you protect my child on the way to school?* If you worry about your children being injured on the playground, you could make another request to protect them during recess time: *Dear Sha's Golden Healing Ball, my children are playing at school. Please do not let them fall down. Take good care of them. Thank you.* Sha's Golden Healing Ball *will* protect your children.

As with all the techniques presented in this book, remember to thank the holy beings, mantras, and spiritual healing tools from whom you have requested a healing and protection blessing. Expressing your gratitude and appreciation is a most important spiritual courtesy that you must never forget to observe.

Healing on a Grand Scale

Pollution is a huge problem for Mother Earth and the whole universe. Virtually every country generates toxic chemicals, wastes, and other forms of pollution. Garbage, noxious emissions, chemical effluent, waste from factories, contaminated waterways, and so on are all different forms of energy. Billions of dollars have been spent by governments, corporations, and researchers on studying, creating, and complying with environmental regulations enacted around the world. Why, then, is there still no solution? Why does poisoning of the Earth continue? Can the damage be undone? The answer is beyond most people's thinking. The true solution for pollution will be on the soul level.

Physicists understand the Law of the Conservation of Energy, which explains that energy never disappears, nor can it be destroyed. Energy merely changes from one form to another. From this perspective, pollution or waste can be understood as atrophy, as just another form of energy. Just as urine and feces are the wastes or atrophy of the body, pollution is the waste or atrophy of the Earth. However, put the atrophy of human waste on plants and vegetables and it becomes fertilizer, providing nutrients for plant organisms. In this way, atrophy is transformed into negative atrophy, or nutrients.

The human organism does not like atrophy, but it likes negative atrophy. Cancer cells are the result of atrophy. They are part of the body's waste, but they can be transformed. For example, if you have lung cancer, you can use the One Hand Near, One Hand Far healing technique to heal it. Repeatedly chant the healing numbers three and nine in Chinese (*san jiu*, pronounced "sahn joe") and visualize light dissipating from your lungs. In your mind's eye, move the light from your lungs to your lower abdomen. Visualize the light flowing, and the energy will move. The energy around the cancer cells in the lungs is atrophy, yet when that energy is moved to the lower abdomen it turns into negative atrophy, which is a nutrient for the foundational energy centers in the lower abdomen. What was once negative becomes positive. Yin turns into yang. Cancer cells transform back into normal cells.

The atrophy of pollution can also be transformed by using Soul Power. Just apply Say Hello Healing and ask powerful mantras, holy beings, corporations, and the pollution itself to heal the pollution problem. However, it will take a great number of souls — the souls of the pollution, Heaven, the stars, the Divine, healing angels, Buddhas, saints, as well as many earthly souls — to transform pollution on a global scale. When the time is right, all the necessary souls in the universe will join together to transform the waste and atrophy of pollution into negative atrophy, or nourishment for the planet. Be patient. Healing will come when the time is right for this global transformation.

Using the Four Power Techniques to Heal Common Ailments

You have now learned the key theories and techniques of Soul Mind Body Medicine. You have received the simple, sacred wisdom and knowledge that are the foundation and core of this new medicine for the twenty-first century: Soul Power and Say Hello Healing. You have been taught practical exercises for developing Mind Power. You have been offered some of the most powerful healing mantras of our time and from ancient history. You have seen how to combine the Four Power Techniques in One-Minute Healing, Universal Meditation, and other simple healing methods. You have been given specific healing protocols for losing weight, recovering from cancer, and for balancing emotions.

This chapter is one of the most practical in this book. It shows you how to use the Four Power Techniques of Soul Mind Body Medicine to heal more than one hundred common ailments. It is a healing handbook that brings the application of Soul Mind Body Medicine to the most specific and concrete level. Use it often — for yourself, your loved ones, and your colleagues — as the need arises. Use it daily to heal soul, mind, and body.

The common ailments included in this chapter, in this order, are: conditions of the head, conditions of the eyes, conditions of the nose, conditions of the mouth, conditions of the ears, conditions of the neck, conditions of the lungs, colds, conditions of the heart, conditions of the spleen and stomach, conditions of the liver and gallbladder, conditions of the kidneys and bladder, conditions of the lower abdomen, feminine conditions, conditions of the blood vessels, conditions of the bones and joints, and conditions of the skin.

For each condition, you will find a photograph demonstrating the applicable Body Power position. This is followed by brief descriptions of the recommended Body Power, Soul Power, Sound Power, and Mind Power techniques. In the next few pages, I will provide some additional wisdom and knowledge to deepen your understanding of the Four Power Techniques of Soul Mind Body Medicine. Then, you will be able to follow the specific examples with confidence to serve yourself and others. The Four Power Techniques of Soul Mind Body Medicine are honored to serve you.

BODY POWER

The Body Power technique used for almost all the ailments in this chapter is the One Hand Near, One Hand Far healing technique.

To review, the One Hand Near, One Hand Far healing technique is based on the principle that high density or pressure flows to low density or pressure naturally. The Near Hand is placed four to seven inches from the area of the body that has high energy density, while the Far Hand is placed fifteen to twenty inches from the body, creating a difference in density or pressure in the energy fields between the hands and the body.

The energy field between the Near Hand and the body will have relatively high density. The energy field between the Far Hand and the body will have relatively low density. Energy will flow naturally from the higher-density field to the lower-density field. Excess or blocked energy in the area the Near Hand faces will move away, removing the energy blockage in that area and promoting healing of the pain, inflammation, emotional imbalance, cysts, tumors, cancer, or other ailments resulting from that blockage.

The excess energy moves to the area the Far Hand faces. Generally, this is the lower abdomen, the location of the Lower Dan Tian, a foundational energy center that always benefits from more energy. If you have pain in one area and weakness in another, you can place the Near Hand facing the painful area and the Far Hand facing the weak area, moving the excess energy away from the painful area to boost the insufficient energy in the weak area.

You can enhance the One Hand Near, One Hand Far technique by pointing your fingers in the direction in which you want energy to flow. For example, for a headache or sore throat, when you want blocked energy to flow *down* from the painful area, you can point the fingertips of your Near Hand *downward*. This will reinforce the movement of energy from the head or throat to the lower abdomen. Don't point your Near Hand fingers up at the head or throat, because doing so will work against the desired downward flow of light and energy.

On the other hand, if you have a degenerative weakness in the brain, such as poor memory, then you want to bring energy *up* from the lower part of your body to your head. The Near Hand would face a kidney or the Snow Mountain Area (the lower back), and the Far Hand would face your head. Point the fingertips of the Near Hand *upward*, because you want to send light and energy up.

The One Hand Near, One Hand Far healing technique is very simple, but all the same, pay great attention to it. Because of your hand positions, this is a very visual technique enabling you to see healing in action. This Body Power technique alone can bring immediate healing benefits by reducing or removing energy and spiritual blockages.

Give the One Hand Near, One Hand Far healing technique a try the next time you have a headache or catch a cold. It only takes a few minutes. Practice it five times a day. You will be amazed at how much improvement you will notice. The next day, you could notice a major difference. Don't think that because it is so simple this technique is not powerful. It is one of Master Guo's greatest contributions to healing.

SOUL POWER

Soul Power is the most simple, but the most essential, of the Four Power Techniques. The use of Soul Power follows the healing formula introduced in chapter 2. There are five simple components to this formula:

1. Say hello: *Dear soul, mind, and body of my _____ ,*

2. Give love: *I love you.*

3. Make an affirmation: *You have the power to heal yourself.*

4. Give an order: *Do a good job!*

5. Express gratitude and courtesy: *Thank you.*

Remember this formula for every self-healing and healing situation. In this chapter we will follow this formula consistently by first saying hello to the inner souls of our area of sickness and our hands. Although you can be creative and flexible in how you say hello, never forget to speak to your inner souls first.

SOUND POWER

In previous chapters, I introduced various Sound Power tools, including powerful mantras such as *Weng Ar Hong* and *San San Jiu Liu Ba Yao Wu* (3396815) in chapter 4, and various number sounds in Chinese in chapter 6. All Sound Power tools work in part because sound vibrates the body. Indeed, sound is vibration. Specific sounds stimulate cellular vibration in specific parts of the body. To review 3396815, you can refer to the detailed explanation and diagram (see figure 9, p. 158) in chapter 4.

When you repeat the sounds of the numbers one through eleven in Chinese, you will feel the vibration in different parts of your body. If your Third Eye is open, you can see the vibration in your body. For example, the number one, *yi*, which is pronounced "ee," vibrates the brain and head. You can confirm this easily. Put one palm against your head and chant *ee, ee, ee, ee, ee, ee, ee, ee.* Feel the vibration in your head.

Most of the examples in this chapter use a combination of two number sounds to transfer energy from one part of the body to another. Sometimes, a combination of three number sounds is used. The resulting transfer of energy supports and reinforces the transfer of energy promoted by the One Hand Near, One Hand Far healing method described above and the Mind Power visualization of light described below. Any one of the Four Power Techniques alone is a powerful healing tool, but it is much more powerful to use the Four Power Techniques together, particularly with the inclusion of Soul Power.

In some examples, a single number sound is used to build and develop energy in a specific organ or area of the body. This typically occurs in healing for degenerative illnesses, which are due to an insufficiency of energy and cellular vibration. The numbers one through eleven in Chinese, their pronunciations, and the areas of the body that they stimulate are shown in table 7.

Table 7. Number Sounds 1 to 11

Number	Chinese Word	Pronunciation	Area Stimulated
1	*yi* or *yao*	"ee" or "yow"	head, brain
2	*ar*	"ar"	heart
3	*san*	"sahn"	chest, lungs
4	*si*	"sih"	esophagus
5	*wu*	"woo"	stomach, spleen
6	*liu*	"lew"	ribs
7	*chi*	"chee"	liver
8	*ba*	"bah"	navel
9	*jiu*	"joe"	lower abdomen
10	*shi*	"shih"	anus
11	*shiyi*	"shih-ee"	limbs, extremities

Use the number sounds as indicated for each specific condition. Also remember that for any condition, you can always chant *San San Jiu Liu Ba Yao Wu* (3396815) or use Sha's Golden Healing Ball as the Sound Power technique. You can invoke these two divine treasures to serve your healing at any time.

MIND POWER

The major Mind Power technique is to visualize golden or white light. When you want to transfer energy, visualize light moving through the body from one area — usually the area the Near Hand faces — to another, usually the area the Far Hand faces. The Far Hand often faces the lower abdomen or Lower Dan Tian, as explained above.

Visualizing light is better than visualizing energy. Moving the light within your body, typically to the Lower Dan Tian, is better than radiating light and energy to the universe. We want to save the blocked energy and put it to better use. Blocked energy is not bad energy; rather, it is a positive force that, once it is moved from the area of blockage, can be used beneficially elsewhere.

When insufficient energy, characterized by weakness, fatigue, and degenerative changes, is the cause of illness, visualize light coming in from the universe to concentrate and intensify in the organ or area needing more energy. Never visualize or think about sending energy or light out. You will drain yourself if you do. Do not send light or energy out of your body, whether you are healing yourself or others.

There is always room for creativity and flexibility. For example, it is perfectly okay if you want to visualize rainbow light instead of golden or white light.

SOME GENERAL INSTRUCTIONS

It is best to practice all the healing techniques of Soul Mind Body Medicine in a calm, relaxed state and in a calm, relaxed environment. A calm, relaxed state will open your soul, mind, systems, organs, and cells to benefit fully from the healing. It will itself promote balance in your cellular vibration and internal flow of energy. A calm, relaxed environment will allow you to open further and to focus fully on the healing. Here are a few more pointers to help get you on your way to healing.

One-Hand Healing Technique

To address several of the conditions in this chapter, we use the One-Hand Healing technique, introduced in chapter 6 as a Body Power technique for group healing and remote healing (see figure 25, p. 167). For self-healing, the One-Hand Healing technique is very simple:

- Point one hand at the affected area from ten to twenty inches away. (In some cases, the hand is held nearer than ten inches away. Also, in some cases the hand is not pointing.)

- Visualize bright golden or white light glowing, radiating in the area. Visualize the area as unblocked, translucent, and healthy.

- Chant *San San Jiu Liu Ba Yao Wu* (3396815) or the specific number sound(s) noted for the condition.

- As with the conditions using the One Hand Near, One Hand Far healing technique, practice three to five minutes per time, three to five times per day.

Length of Practice

Generally speaking, with all these techniques, practice three to five minutes per time, three to five times per day. It is not necessary to spend more time for each healing. However, if you have chronic pain, chronic illness, or a life-threatening illness such as cancer, use Sha's Golden Healing Ball together with the Four Power Techniques. Say "hello" to and ask Sha's Golden Healing Ball to rotate in your area of illness. For serious conditions, you can continue to do the healing for a full half hour or even an entire hour, with no problem.

CONDITIONS OF THE HEAD

Dizziness

BODY POWER. Near Hand: side of the head; Far Hand: upper, opposite side of the head

SOUL POWER. *Dear soul, mind, and body of my head, I love you. You have the power to heal yourself. Dear soul, mind, and body of my hands,* yi, *and light, I love you all. You have the power to heal me. Do a good job. Thank you. Thank you. Thank you.*

SOUND POWER. Chant *yi* (one, pronounced "ee").

MIND POWER. Visualize bright golden or white light glowing in the brain.

Notes

Alternate the hand positions to complete this procedure. Dizziness is commonly caused by poor capillary circulation in the head.

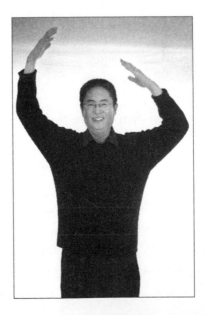

Headache, Parietal

(crown of the head)

BODY POWER. Near Hand: over the crown of the head; Far Hand: lower abdomen (Lower Dan Tian)

SOUL POWER. *Dear soul, mind, and body of my head, I love you. You have the power to heal yourself. Dear soul, mind, and body of my hands,* yi-jiu, *and light, I love you all. You have the power to heal me. Do a good job. Thank you. Thank you. Thank you.*

SOUND POWER. Chant *yi-jiu* (one-nine, pronounced "ee-joe").

MIND POWER. Visualize bright golden or white light flowing from the crown of the head to the lower abdomen.

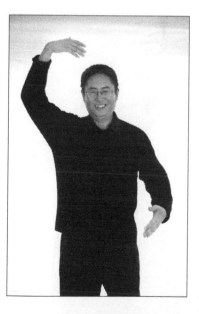

Headache, Frontal

(forehead)

BODY POWER. Near Hand: forehead or the point midway between the eyebrows (Yin Tang acupuncture point); Far Hand: lower abdomen (Lower Dan Tian)

SOUL POWER. *Dear soul, mind, and body of my head, I love you. You have the power to heal yourself. Dear soul, mind, and body of my hands,* yi-jiu, *and light, I love you all. You have the power to heal me. Do a good job. Thank you. Thank you. Thank you.*

SOUND POWER. Chant *yi-jiu* (one-nine, pronounced "ee-joe").

MIND POWER. Visualize bright golden or white light flowing from the forehead to the lower abdomen.

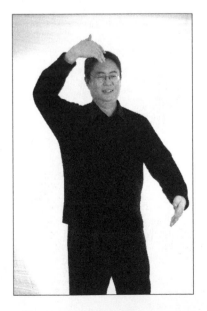

Headache, Temporal

(temple)

BODY POWER. Near Hand: four fingertips point down toward the temple; Far Hand: lower abdomen (Lower Dan Tian)

SOUL POWER. *Dear soul, mind, and body of my head, I love you. You have the power to heal yourself. Dear soul, mind, and body of my hands,* yi-jiu, *and light, I love you all. You have the power to heal me. Do a good job. Thank you. Thank you. Thank you.*

SOUND POWER. Chant *yi-jiu* (one-nine, pronounced "ee-joe").

MIND POWER. Visualize bright golden or white light flowing from the temple area to the lower abdomen.

Notes

Do not point up with the Near Hand. Alternate hands if you have pain in both temples.

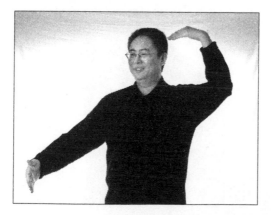

Headache, Suboccipital

(base of the neck)

BODY POWER. Near Hand: four fingertips point at the back of the neck; Far Hand: lower abdomen (Lower Dan Tian)

SOUL POWER. *Dear soul, mind, and body of my head and neck, I love you. You have the power to heal yourselves. Dear soul, mind, and body of my hands,* yi-jiu, *and light, I love you all. You have the power to heal me. Do a good job. Thank you. Thank you. Thank you.*

SOUND POWER. Chant *yi-jiu* (one-nine, pronounced "ee-joe").

MIND POWER. Visualize bright golden or white light flowing from the back of the head to the lower abdomen.

Notes

This condition is commonly caused by holding tension in the neck.

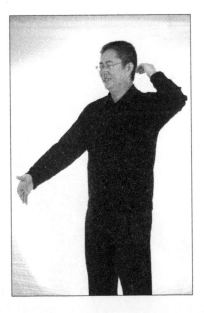

High Blood Pressure

high systolic, high diastolic
(hypertension: high systolic)

BODY POWER. Near Hand: over the crown of the head or facing the forehead; Far Hand: lower abdomen (Lower Dan Tian)

SOUL POWER. *Dear soul, mind, and body of my head and my circulatory system, I love you. You have the power to heal yourselves. Dear soul, mind, and body of my hands, yi-jiu, and light, I love you all. You have the power to heal me. Do a good job. Thank you. Thank you. Thank you.*

SOUND POWER. Chant *yi-jiu* (one-nine, pronounced "ee-joe").

MIND POWER. Visualize bright golden or white light flowing from the head to the lower abdomen.

Notes

Follow this procedure if you have high systolic and high diastolic blood pressure, or if you have high systolic and normal diastolic blood pressure.

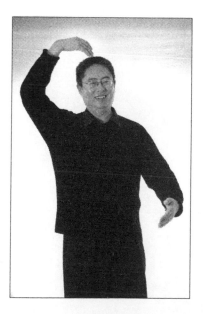

High Blood Pressure

normal systolic, high diastolic
(hypertension: high diastolic)

BODY POWER. Near Hand: heart or the middle of the chest (Message Center); Far Hand: lower abdomen (Lower Dan Tian)

SOUL POWER. *Dear soul, mind, and body of my circulatory system, I love you. You have the power to heal yourselves. Dear soul, mind, and body of my hands, ar-jiu, and light, I love you all. You have the power to heal me. Do a good job. Thank you. Thank you. Thank you.*

SOUND POWER. Chant *ar-jiu* (two-nine, pronounced "ar-joe").

MIND POWER. Visualize bright golden or white light flowing from the heart to the lower abdomen.

Notes

Follow this procedure if you have normal systolic and high diastolic blood pressure. High blood pressure is caused by too much energy in the heart.

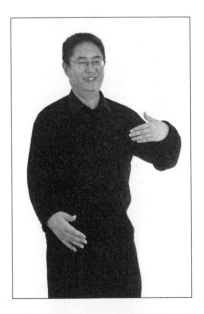

Low Blood Pressure

(hypotension)

BODY POWER. Near Hand: lower abdomen (Lower Dan Tian); Far Hand: crown of the head, the forehead, or the point midway between the eyebrows (Yin Tang acupuncture point)

SOUL POWER. *Dear soul, mind, and body of my Lower Dan Tian and my circulatory system, I love you. You have the power to heal yourselves. Dear soul, mind, and body of my hands,* ar-jiu, *and light, I love you all. You have the power to heal me. Do a good job. Thank you. Thank you. Thank you.*

SOUND POWER. Chant *jiu-yi* (nine-one, pronounced "joe-ee").

MIND POWER. Visualize bright golden or white light flowing from the lower abdomen to the head.

Notes

Do not use this technique if you have glaucoma.

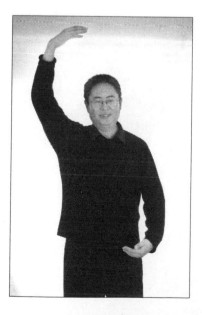

Stroke

(left-side paralysis)

BODY POWER. Near Hand: right palm faces, or the fingers of the right hand point to, the right side of the brain; Far Hand: left hand faces the left side of the body

SOUL POWER. *Dear soul, mind, and body of my brain, my nervous system, and my circulatory system, I love you. You have the power to heal yourselves. Dear soul, mind, and body of my hands, yi-jiu, and light, I love you all. You have the power to heal me. Do a good job. Thank you. Thank you. Thank you.*

SOUND POWER. Chant *yi-jiu* (one-nine, pronounced "ee-joe").

MIND POWER. Visualize bright golden or white light flowing from the right side of the head to the left side of the body.

Notes

Paralysis on the left side of the body is due to a hemorrhage or blood clot (energy blockage) on the right side of the brain. Be sure to position the hands correctly; reversing hand positions may worsen the condition.

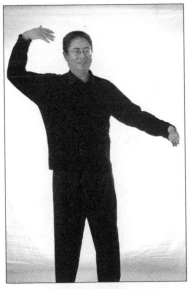

Stroke

(right-side paralysis)

BODY POWER. Near Hand: left palm faces, or the fingers of the left hand point to, the left side of the brain; Far Hand: right hand faces the right side of the body

SOUL POWER. *Dear soul, mind, and body of my brain, my nervous system, and my circulatory system, I love you. You have the power to heal yourselves. Dear soul, mind, and body of my hands, yi-jiu, and light, I love you all. You have the power to heal me. Do a good job. Thank you. Thank you. Thank you.*

SOUND POWER. Chant *yi-jiu* (one-nine, pronounced "ee-joe").

MIND POWER. Visualize bright golden or white light flowing from the left side of the head to the right side of the body.

Notes

Paralysis on the right side of the body is due to a hemorrhage or blood clot (energy blockage) on the left side of the brain. Be sure to position the hands correctly; reversing the hand positions may worsen the condition.

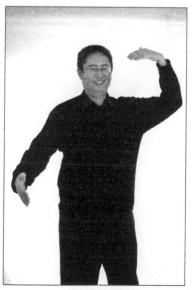

Hardening of the Brain Arteries

(cerebral arteriosclerosis)

BODY POWER. Near Hand: any side of the head; shake the hand rapidly; Far Hand: lower abdomen (Lower Dan Tian)

SOUL POWER. *Dear soul, mind, and body of my brain and my circulatory system, I love you. You have the power to heal yourselves. Dear soul, mind, and body of my hands,* yi-jiu, *and light, I love you all. You have the power to heal me. Do a good job. Thank you. Thank you. Thank you. Thank you.*

SOUND POWER. Chant *yi-jiu* (one-nine, pronounced "ee-joe").

MIND POWER. Visualize bright golden or white light flowing from the head to the lower abdomen or radiating throughout the brain.

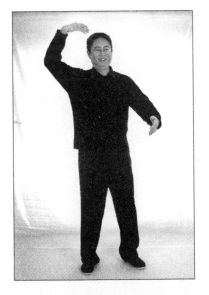

Brain Tumor

(or cancer)

BODY POWER. Near Hand: point and shake the middle finger at the tumor from two inches away; Far Hand: lower abdomen (Lower Dan Tian)

SOUL POWER. *Dear soul, mind, and body of my tumor cells (or cancer cells), I love you. You've gone in the wrong direction. You have the power to heal yourselves. You have the power to turn back to normal cells. Dear soul, mind, and body of my hands, yi-jiu, and light, I love you all. You have the power to heal me. Do a good job. Thank you. Thank you. Thank you.*

SOUND POWER. Chant *yi-jiu* (one-nine, pronounced "ee-joe").

MIND POWER. Visualize bright golden or white light flowing from the area of the tumor to the lower abdomen.

Notes

Don't think about the tumor itself. Instead, think that the area of the tumor is healthy and glowing with light. Send your greatest love to the tumor or cancer cells, to all your brain cells.

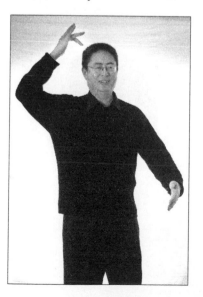

Senility, Dementia, Alzheimer's Disease

Step 1 of 2

BODY POWER. Place both hands behind you, with palms facing the Snow Mountain Area.

SOUL POWER. *Dear soul, mind, and body of my Snow Mountain Area, I love you. You have the power to boost your energy. Dear soul, mind, and body of my hands,* jiu, *and light, I love you all. You have the power to boost my Snow Mountain Area. Do a good job. Thank you. Thank you. Thank you.*

SOUND POWER. Chant *jiu* (nine, pronounced "joe").

MIND POWER. Visualize a snow-covered mountain in the Snow Mountain Area. Imagine a very hot, strong sun shining on the mountain. The snow is melting, and energy in the form of steam rises and flows to any part of your body that you wish to nourish or heal.

Notes

Senility and Alzheimer's disease are a result of weak kidney function. The solution is to build the Snow Mountain Area to build kidney energy. Then, send the kidney energy up to nourish the brain.

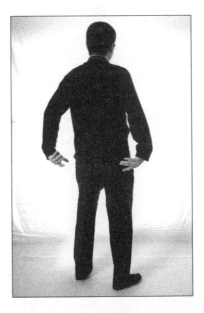

Senility, Dementia, Alzheimer's Disease

Step 2 of 2

BODY POWER. Near Hand: a kidney or the Snow Mountain Area; Far Hand: over the crown of the head

SOUL POWER. *Dear soul, mind, and body of my brain, I love you. You have the power to heal yourselves. Dear soul, mind, and body of my hands, jiu-yi, and light, I love you all. You have the power to heal me. Do a good job. Thank you. Thank you. Thank you.*

SOUND POWER. Chant *jiu-yi* (nine-one, pronounced "joe-ee").

MIND POWER. Visualize bright golden or white light flowing from the Snow Mountain Area up the spinal column to the top of the head (Bai Hui acupuncture point) and nourishing the brain.

Notes

Do not use this technique if you have high blood pressure, a brain tumor, or brain cancer.

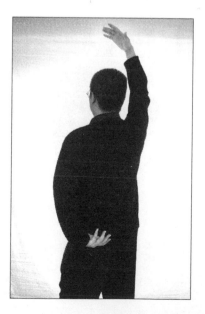

195

Hyperactivity

(in children)

BODY POWER. Use the One-Hand Healing technique for the child. Pat the child's head or shake one hand over the crown of his or her head, about two inches above.

SOUL POWER. *Dear soul, mind, and body of Alice's* [for example] *brain, I love you. You have the power to heal yourselves. Dear soul, mind, and body of my hand,* yi, *and light, I love you all. You have the power to heal Alice's brain. Do a good job. Thank you. Thank you. Thank you.*

SOUND POWER. Chant *yi* (one, pronounced "ee").

MIND POWER. Visualize bright golden or white light from the universe flowing into the child's brain. Think of the child as clear-minded and intelligent.

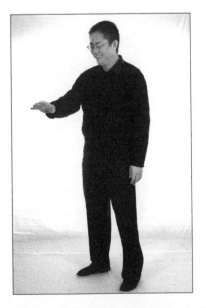

CONDITIONS OF THE EYES

Nearsightedness

(recent onset)

BODY POWER. Near Hand: right palm faces the liver diagonally; shake the right hand; Far Hand: forehead or the point midway between the eyebrows (Yin Tang acupuncture point); if the liver is weak, the left hand faces the lower abdomen (Lower Dan Tian)

SOUL POWER. *Dear soul, mind, and body of my eyes and liver, I love you. You have the power to heal yourselves. Dear soul, mind, and body of my hands,* chi-yi, *and light, I love you all. You have the power to heal me. Do a good job. Thank you. Thank you. Thank you.*

SOUND POWER. Chant *chi-yi* (seven-one, pronounced "chee-ee"); *chi-jiu* (seven-nine, pronounced "chee-joe") if the left hand faces the lower abdomen.

MIND POWER. Visualize bright golden or white light flowing from the liver to the point midway between the eyebrows.

Notes

"The liver opens on the eyes." In traditional Chinese medicine, the eye is connected to the liver meridian; the eyes often reflect the health of the liver.

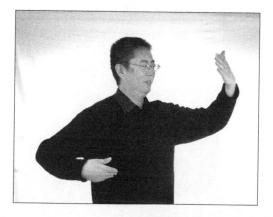

Cataracts

BODY POWER. Use the One-Hand Healing technique. Cup the fingertips (as if you were holding an eyeball) at a distance of four to seven inches from the eye.

SOUL POWER. *Dear soul, mind, and body of my eyes, I love you. You have the power to heal yourselves. Dear soul, mind, and body of my hand, yi, and light, I love you all. You have the power to heal me. Do a good job. Thank you. Thank you. Thank you.*

SOUND POWER. Chant *yi* (one, pronounced "ee").

MIND POWER. Visualize bright golden or white light dissipating from the eye. Imagine the surface-layer cells of the eyeball vibrating. See the eyeball as clean, shiny, and clear.

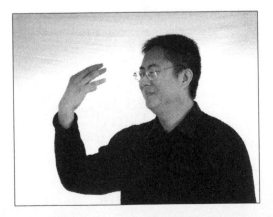

Glaucoma

BODY POWER. Near Hand: forehead or the point midway between the eyebrows (Yin Tang accupuncture point); Far Hand: palm faces the liver diagonally

SOUL POWER. *Dear soul, mind, and body of my eyes and liver, I love you. You have the power to heal yourselves. Dear soul, mind, and body of my hands,* yi-chi, *and light, I love you all. You have the power to heal me. Do a good job. Thank you. Thank you. Thank you.*

SOUND POWER. Chant *yi-chi* (one-seven, pronounced "ee-chee").

MIND POWER. Visualize bright golden or white light flowing from the point between the eyebrows to the liver.

Notes

Do not point the Near Hand directly at the eyes, since too much energy can harm their delicate tissues.

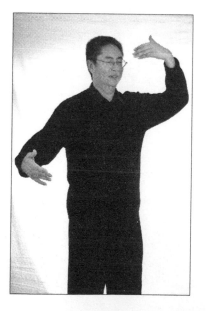

Retinal Atrophy

BODY POWER. Near Hand: center of the lower back (Snow Mountain Area); Far Hand: forehead or the midpoint between the eyebrows (Yin Tang acupuncture point)

SOUL POWER. *Dear soul, mind, and body of my eyes, I love you. You have the power to heal yourselves. Dear soul, mind, and body of my hands,* jiu-yi, *and light, I love you all. You have the power to heal me. Do a good job. Thank you. Thank you. Thank you.*

SOUND POWER. Chant *jiu-yi* (nine-one, pronounced "joe-ee").

MIND POWER. Visualize bright golden or white light flowing from the lower back (Snow Mountain Area) to the point between the eyebrows.

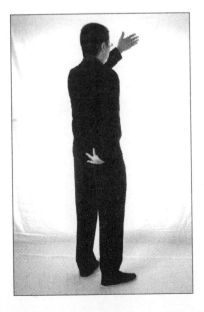

Sties and Sore, Irritated Eyes

(opthalmia, conjunctivitis)

BODY POWER. Near Hand: forehead or midpoint between the eyebrows (Yin Tang acupuncture point); Far Hand: lower abdomen (Lower Dan Tian)

SOUL POWER. *Dear soul, mind, and body of my eyes, I love you. You have the power to heal yourselves. Dear soul, mind, and body of my hands,* yi-jiu, *and light, I love you all. You have the power to heal me. Do a good job. Thank you. Thank you. Thank you.*

SOUND POWER. Chant *yi-jiu* (one-nine, pronounced "ee-joe").

MIND POWER. Visualize bright golden or white light flowing from the point between the eyebrows to the lower abdomen.

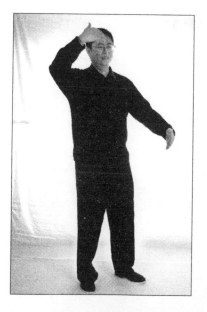

Chronic Tearing

(dacryocystitis)

BODY POWER. Using the One-Hand Healing technique, hold the palm steady at a distance of ten to fifteen inches from the affected eye(s).

SOUL POWER. *Dear soul, mind, and body of my eyes, I love you. You have the power to heal yourselves. Dear soul, mind, and body of my hand,* yi, *and light, I love you all. You have the power to heal me. Do a good job. Thank you. Thank you. Thank you.*

SOUND POWER. Chant *yi* (one, pronounced "ee").

MIND POWER. Stare at the palm of your hand with both eyes and without blinking to induce the eyes to start watering and tearing.

Notes

Chronic tearing is the result of blocked tear ducts. Not blinking will stimulate tear production, helping to cleanse and remove blockages from the tear ducts.

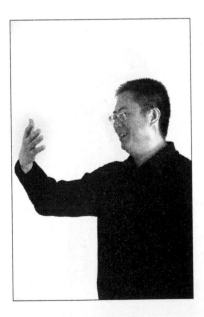

Seeing Spots or Lines

(floaters)

BODY POWER. Near Hand: lower back/kidneys (Snow Mountain Area); Far Hand: eyes

SOUL POWER. *Dear soul, mind, and body of my eyes and kidneys, I love you. You have the power to heal yourselves. Dear soul, mind, and body of my hands,* jiu-yi, *and light, I love you all. You have the power to heal me. Do a good job. Thank you. Thank you. Thank you.*

SOUND POWER. Chant *jiu-yi* (nine-one, pronounced "joe-ee").

MIND POWER. Visualize bright golden or white light flowing from the kidney area (Snow Mountain Area) to the point midway between the eyebrows (Yin Tang acupuncture point).

Notes

If the kidneys are weak, develop more kidney energy first by following the procedure for Kidney Inflammation (p. 266).

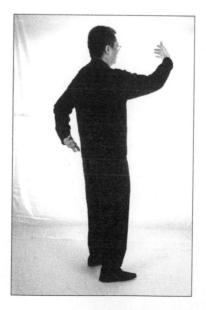

Crossed Eyes

(strabismus)

BODY POWER. Put the backs of your hands together, and gradually pull them apart in front of your eyes.

SOUL POWER. *Dear soul, mind, and body of my eyes, I love you. You have the power to heal yourselves. Dear soul, mind, and body of my hands,* yi, *and light, I love you all. You have the power to heal me. Do a good job. Thank you. Thank you. Thank you.*

SOUND POWER. Chant *yi* (one, pronounced "ee").

MIND POWER. Visualize the eyes separating and aligning properly.

Notes

It takes time to correct crossed eyes, so repeat this procedure many times. If only one eye is crossed, move only one hand as if you were aligning the eye. For walled eyes (the opposite of crossed eyes), start with the backs of the hands head-width apart, and slowly bring them together.

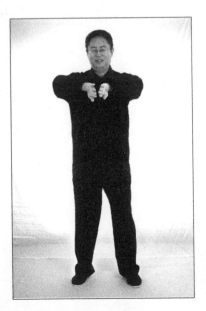 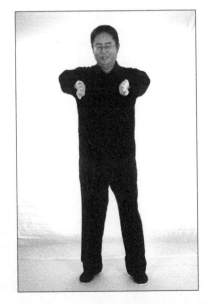

CONDITIONS OF THE NOSE

Congestion in One Nostril

(nasal sinusitis and rhinitis)

Step 1 of 2

BODY POWER. Using the One-Hand Healing technique, shake your hand at the blocked nostril.

SOUL POWER. *Dear soul, mind, and body of my nostril, I love you. You have the power to heal yourself. Dear soul, mind, and body of my hand,* san-wu, *and light, I love you all. You have the power to heal me. Do a good job. Thank you. Thank you. Thank you.*

SOUND POWER. Chant *san-wu* (three-five, pronounced "sahn-woo").

MIND POWER. Visualize bright golden or white light flowing out of the blocked nostril.

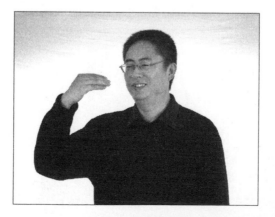

Congestion in One Nostril

(nasal sinusitis and rhinitis)

Step 2 of 2

BODY POWER. Using the One-Hand Healing technique, point an index finger at the blocked nostril from about two inches away.

SOUL POWER. *Dear soul, mind, and body of my nostril, I love you. You have the power to heal yourselves. Dear soul, mind, and body of my hand,* yi-san-wu-jiu, *and light, I love you all. You have the power to heal me. Do a good job. Thank you. Thank you. Thank you.*

SOUND POWER. Chant *yi-san-wu-jiu* (one-three-five-nine, pronounced "ee-sahn-woo-joe").

MIND POWER. Visualize bright golden or white light flowing from the blocked nostril, through the lungs, down through the stomach, and into the Lower Dan Tian (lower abdomen).

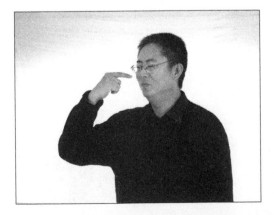

Congestion in Both Nostrils

(nasal sinusitis and rhinitis)

Step 1 of 2

BODY POWER. Near Hand: spread the index and the middle fingers in a V pointing at both nostrils; Far Hand: lower abdomen (Lower Dan Tian); shake the hand

SOUL POWER. *Dear soul, mind, and body of my nostrils, I love you. You have the power to heal yourselves. Dear soul, mind, and body of my hands, ar, and light, I love you all. You have the power to heal me. Do a good job. Thank you. Thank you. Thank you.*

SOUND POWER. Chant *ar* (two, pronounced "ar").

MIND POWER. Visualize bright golden or white light glowing in the nose.

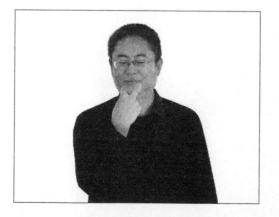

Congestion in Both Nostrils
(nasal sinusitis and rhinitis)

Step 2 of 2

BODY POWER. Near Hand: from about two or three inches away, point the index finger and the middle finger at both sides of the point midway between the eyebrows (Yin Tang acupuncture point); the fingers should point slightly downward; Far Hand: stomach

SOUL POWER. *Dear soul, mind, and body of my nostrils, I love you. You have the power to heal yourselves. Dear soul, mind, and body of my hands,* yi-san-wu, *and light, I love you all. You have the power to heal me. Do a good job. Thank you. Thank you. Thank you.*

SOUND POWER. Chant *yi-san-wu* (one-three-five, pronounced "ee-sahn-woo").

MIND POWER. Visualize bright golden or white light flowing from the nose through the lungs to the stomach.

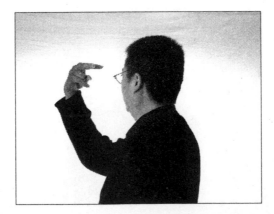

Stuffy or Runny Nose

(due to colds, allergies, or inflammation)

BODY POWER. Near Hand: middle of the chest, above the nipples; Far Hand: side of the body, at chest level

SOUL POWER. *Dear soul, mind, and body of my nose, I love you. You have the power to heal yourselves. Dear soul, mind, and body of my hands,* san-wu, *and light, I love you all. You have the power to heal me. Do a good job. Thank you. Thank you. Thank you.*

SOUND POWER. Chant *san-wu* (three-five, pronounced "sahn-woo").

MIND POWER. Visualize bright golden or white light flowing from the lungs down to the stomach.

Notes

This condition is due to energy not flowing properly in the lungs.

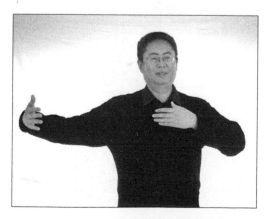

Stuffy Nose and Sinuses with Fever

(acute rhinitis and sinusitis)

BODY POWER. Near Hand: chest area; Far Hand: extend the arm (at chest level) with the fingers pointing straight ahead and away from the body

SOUL POWER. *Dear soul, mind, and body of my nose, I love you. You have the power to heal yourselves. Dear soul, mind, and body of my hands,* san-wu, *and light, I love you all. You have the power to heal me. Do a good job. Thank you. Thank you. Thank you.*

SOUND POWER. Chant *san-wu* (three-five, pronounced "sahn-woo").

MIND POWER. Visualize bright golden or white light flowing from the lungs down to the stomach.

Notes

Follow this procedure for only two minutes. If you do it longer, you will lose energy, because the fingers are pointing out and directing energy away from the body.

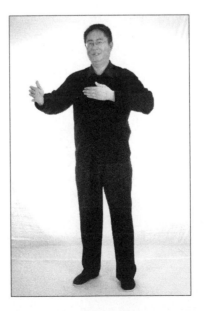

Chronic Postnasal Drip

BODY POWER. Using the One-Hand Healing technique, tilt the palm up slightly, facing the nose or the midpoint between the eyebrows (Yin Tang acupuncture point).

SOUL POWER. *Dear soul, mind, and body of my nose, I love you. You have the power to heal yourselves. Dear soul, mind, and body of my hand,* san-yi, *and light, I love you all. You have the power to heal me. Do a good job. Thank you. Thank you. Thank you.*

SOUND POWER. Chant *san-yi* (three-one, pronounced "sahn-ee").

MIND POWER. Visualize bright golden or white light flowing from the lungs to the nose.

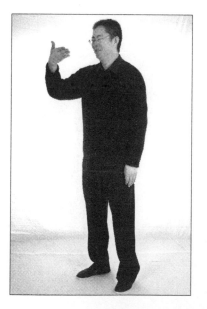

CONDITIONS OF THE MOUTH

Cold Sores or Cankers That Form Cavities

(herpes simplex 1)

BODY POWER. Near Hand: middle finger points to the sore; Far Hand: stomach; angle the hand slightly downward

SOUL POWER. *Dear soul, mind, and body of my cold sore, I love you. You have the power to heal yourselves. Dear soul, mind, and body of my hands,* yi-wu-jiu, *and light, I love you all. You have the power to heal me. Do a good job. Thank you. Thank you. Thank you.*

SOUND POWER. Chant *yi-wu-jiu* (one-five-nine, pronounced "ee-woo-joe").

MIND POWER. Visualize bright golden or white light flowing from the canker, through the stomach, and into the lower abdomen.

Notes

Follow this procedure for cold sores or cankers that form cavities (depressions) around the lips or in the mouth.

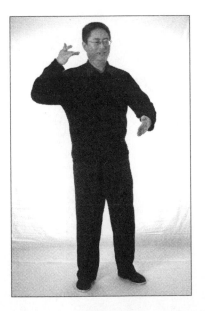

Cold Sores or Cankers That Form Protrusions
(herpes simplex 2)

BODY POWER. Near Hand: stomach; Far Hand: lower abdomen (Lower Dan Tian)

SOUL POWER. *Dear soul, mind, and body of my cold sore, I love you. You have the power to heal yourselves. Dear soul, mind, and body of my hands,* wu-jiu, *and light, I love you all. You have the power to heal me. Do a good job. Thank you. Thank you. Thank you.*

SOUND POWER. Chant *wu-jiu* (five-nine, pronounced "woo-joe").

MIND POWER. Visualize bright golden or white light flowing from the canker, through the stomach, and into the lower abdomen.

Notes

Follow this procedure for cold sores or cankers that form external blisters or moundlike protrusions in and around the mouth.

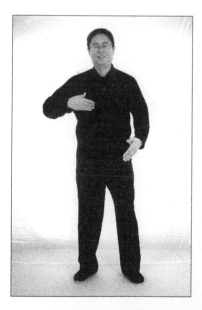

Enlarged Tongue

BODY POWER. Near Hand: right palm, face up, above navel; Far Hand: left palm, face up, below navel

SOUL POWER. *Dear soul, mind, and body of my San Jiao, I love you. You have the power to heal and balance yourselves. Dear soul, mind, and body of my hands, 3396815, and light, I love you all. You have the power to heal me. Do a good job. Thank you. Thank you. Thank you.*

SOUND POWER. Chant *San San Jiu Liu Ba Yao Wu* (3396815, pronounced "sahn sahn joe lew bah yow woo").

MIND POWER. Visualize the numbers 3396815 in a bright golden light ball in your Lower Dan Tian.

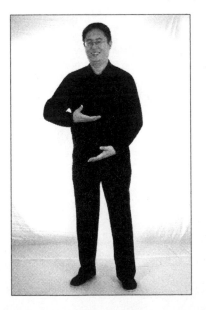

Toothache, Swollen Gums

(gingivitis)

BODY POWER. Near Hand: four fingers point to the affected area; Far Hand: upper abdomen, the stomach

SOUL POWER. *Dear soul, mind, and body of my teeth and gums, I love you. You have the power to heal yourselves. Dear soul, mind, and body of my hands,* yi-wu-jiu, *and light, I love you all. You have the power to heal me. Do a good job. Thank you. Thank you. Thank you.*

SOUND POWER. Chant *yi-wu-jiu* (one-five-nine, pronounced "ee-woo-joe").

MIND POWER. Visualize bright golden or white light flowing from the affected area through the stomach to the lower abdomen.

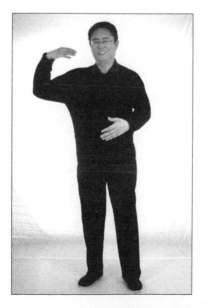

Receding Gums, Periodontal Disease

BODY POWER. Near Hand: lower abdomen (Lower Dan Tian); Far Hand: mouth and gums

SOUL POWER. *Dear soul, mind, and body of my mouth and gums, I love you. You have the power to heal yourselves. Dear soul, mind, and body of my hands, jiu-yi, and light, I love you all. You have the power to heal me. Do a good job. Thank you. Thank you. Thank you.*

SOUND POWER. Chant *jiu-yi* (nine-one, pronounced "joe-ee").

MIND POWER. Visualize light flowing from the lower abdomen to the gums.

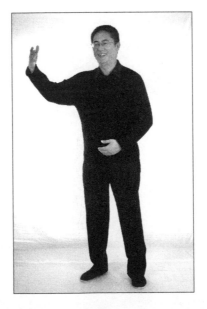

Facial Paralysis with Mouth Twisted to the Left

(Bell's palsy 1)

BODY POWER. Near Hand: left side of the face (the twisted side); Far Hand: right side of the face (the normal side)

SOUL POWER. *Dear soul, mind, and body of my face and nerves, I love you. You have the power to heal yourselves. Dear soul, mind, and body of my hands,* yi, *and light, I love you all. You have the power to heal me. Do a good job. Thank you. Thank you. Thank you.*

SOUND POWER. Chant *yi* (one, pronounced "ee").

MIND POWER. Visualize bright golden or white light flowing from the left (twisted) side of the face to the right (normal) side.

Notes

Left-side disfigurement of the mouth is due to paralysis of the facial nerve on the right side of the face. The normal side is the weak side; the muscles are weak, so send energy to the weak side.

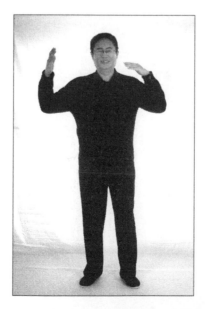

Facial Paralysis with Mouth Twisted to the Right
(Bell's palsy 2)

BODY POWER. Near Hand: right side of the face (the twisted side); Far Hand: left side of the face (the normal side)

SOUL POWER. *Dear soul, mind, and body of my face and nerves, I love you. You have the power to heal yourselves. Dear soul, mind, and body of my hands,* yi, *and light, I love you all. You have the power to heal me. Do a good job. Thank you. Thank you. Thank you.*

SOUND POWER. Chant *yi* (one, pronounced "ee").

MIND POWER. Visualize bright golden or white light flowing from the right (twisted side) of the face to the left (normal) side.

Notes

Right-side disfigurement of the mouth is due to paralysis of the facial nerve on the left side of the face. The normal side is the weak side; the muscles are weak, so send energy to the weak side.

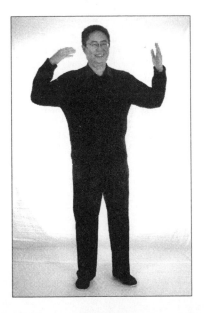

CONDITIONS OF THE EARS

Ringing in the Ears

(tinnitus)

Step 1 of 2

BODY POWER. Near Hand: lower back (Snow Mountain Area); Far Hand: lower back

SOUL POWER. *Dear soul, mind, and body of my Snow Mountain Area, I love you. You have the power to boost yourselves. Dear soul, mind, and body of my hands,* jiu, *and light, I love you all. You have the power to boost my Snow Mountain Area. Do a good job. Thank you. Thank you. Thank you.*

SOUND POWER. Chant *jiu* (nine, pronounced "joe").

MIND POWER. Visualize bright golden or white light radiating in the lower back (Snow Mountain Area).

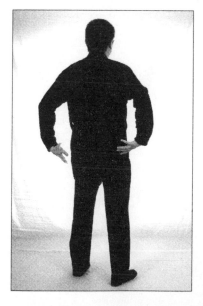

Ringing in the Ears

(tinnitus)

Step 2 of 2

BODY POWER. Near Hand: a kidney; Far Hand: the affected ear

SOUL POWER. *Dear soul, mind, and body of my ear, I love you. You have the power to heal yourselves. Dear soul, mind, and body of my hands,* jiu-yi, *and light, I love you all. You have the power to heal me. Do a good job. Thank you. Thank you. Thank you.*

SOUND POWER. Chant *jiu-yi* (nine-one, pronounced "joe-ee").

MIND POWER. Visualize bright golden or white light flowing from the kidney to the affected ear.

Notes

Tinnitus is caused by weak kidneys. Step 1 boosts energy in the Snow Mountain Area to strengthen kidney chi. This condition, especially if chronic, may take a long time to heal.

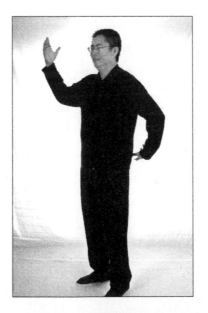

Deafness

BODY POWER. Near Hand: affected ear; Far Hand: opposite ear

SOUL POWER. *Dear soul, mind, and body of my ears, I love you. You have the power to heal yourselves. Dear soul, mind, and body of my hands,* yi, *and light, I love you all. You have the power to heal me. Do a good job. Thank you. Thank you. Thank you.*

SOUND POWER. Chant *yi* (one, pronounced "ee").

MIND POWER. Visualize bright golden or white light flowing from the affected ear to the other ear.

Notes

Alternate hand positions if both ears are affected.

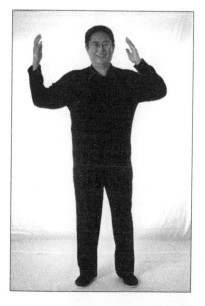

Hearing Loss

(unclear hearing)

BODY POWER. Near Hand: affected ear (cup, but do not touch); Far Hand: opposite ear

SOUL POWER. *Dear soul, mind, and body of my ears, I love you. You have the power to heal yourselves. Dear soul, mind, and body of my hands, yi, and light, I love you all. You have the power to heal me. Do a good job. Thank you. Thank you. Thank you.*

SOUND POWER. Chant *yi* (one, pronounced "ee").

MIND POWER. Visualize bright golden or white light flowing from the affected ear to the other ear.

Notes

Alternate hand positions if both ears are affected. Be persistent, since healing hearing loss is a slow process.

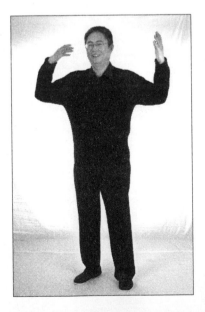

Deafness Caused by Drugs

(iatrogenic deafness)

BODY POWER. Near Hand: affected ear; Far Hand: opposite ear

SOUL POWER. *Dear soul, mind, and body of my ears, I love you. You have the power to heal yourselves. Dear soul, mind, and body of my hands, yi, and light, I love you all. You have the power to heal me. Do a good job. Thank you. Thank you. Thank you.*

SOUND POWER. Chant *yi* (one, pronounced "ee").

MIND POWER. Visualize bright golden or white light flowing from the affected ear to the other ear.

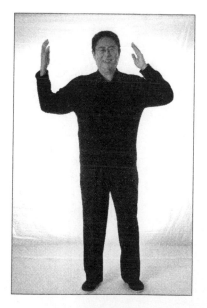

Earache Due to Middle-Ear Inflammation
(otitis media)

BODY POWER. Near Hand: middle finger points to the affected ear; Far Hand: lower abdomen (Lower Dan Tian)

SOUL POWER. *Dear soul, mind, and body of my ear, I love you. You have the power to heal yourselves. Dear soul, mind, and body of my hands, yi-jiu, and light, I love you all. You have the power to heal me. Do a good job. Thank you. Thank you. Thank you.*

SOUND POWER. Chant *yi-jiu* (one-nine, pronounced "ee-joe").

MIND POWER. Visualize bright golden or white light flowing from the affected ear to the lower abdomen.

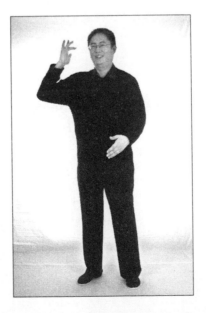

CONDITIONS OF THE NECK

Chronic Sore Throat

(pharyngitis, tonsillitis, laryngitis)

BODY POWER. Using the One-Hand Healing technique, point the fingertips and the thumb at the throat, opening and closing them continuously.

SOUL POWER. *Dear soul, mind, and body of my throat, I love you. You have the power to heal yourselves. Dear soul, mind, and body of my hand,* yi, *and light, I love you all. You have the power to heal me. Do a good job. Thank you. Thank you. Thank you.*

SOUND POWER. Chant *yi* (one, pronounced "ee").

MIND POWER. Visualize the membranes of the throat stretching and loosening, radiating bright golden or white light and becoming smooth and elastic.

Notes

Hoarseness, chronic throat inflammation, and throat membranes that feel rough and tight are symptoms related to the Middle Dan Tian. Consult a physician if the condition lasts for more than two to three weeks, since it may indicate a more serious problem.

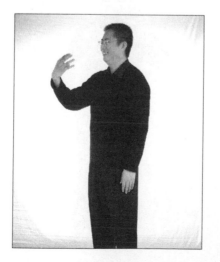

Acute Throat Inflammation

(strep throat)

BODY POWER. Near Hand: point middle finger at the throat; Far Hand: lower abdomen (Lower Dan Tian)

SOUL POWER. *Dear soul, mind, and body of my throat, I love you. You have the power to heal yourself. Dear soul, mind, and body of my hands,* yi-jiu, *and light, I love you all. You have the power to heal me. Do a good job. Thank you. Thank you. Thank you.*

SOUND POWER. Chant *yi-jiu* (one-nine, pronounced "ee-joe").

MIND POWER. Visualize bright golden or white light flowing from the throat to the lower abdomen.

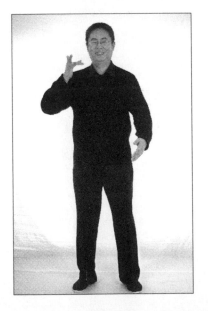

Mumps

(swollen facial or parotid glands)

BODY POWER. Near Hand: stomach; Far Hand: lungs; point hands slightly outward (to reduce the energy of the stomach)

SOUL POWER. *Dear soul, mind, and body of my stomach and lungs, I love you. You have the power to heal yourselves. Dear soul, mind, and body of my hands,* wu-san, *and light, I love you all. You have the power to heal me. Do a good job. Thank you. Thank you. Thank you.*

SOUND POWER. Chant *wu-san* (five-three, pronounced "woo-sahn").

MIND POWER. Visualize bright golden or white light dissipating from the lungs.

Notes

Mumps is due to excess energy in the lungs and stomach. The hand position will remove energy blockages in the lungs and the stomach at the same time. Follow this procedure for only three minutes, and only once or twice a day. Practicing longer can send out too much energy from the body. Do not eat cold foods such as ice cream or drink cold beverages such as ice water.

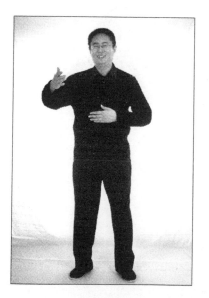

Thyroid Tumor

BODY POWER. Near Hand: point middle finger at the thyroid tumor; Far Hand: right atrium of the heart (the upper left quadrant of the heart in a frontal view)

SOUL POWER. *Dear soul, mind, and body of my thyroid, I love you. You have the power to heal yourselves. Dear soul, mind, and body of my hands,* yi-ar, *and light, I love you all. You have the power to heal me. Do a good job. Thank you. Thank you. Thank you.*

SOUND POWER. Chant *yi-ar* (one-two, pronounced "ee-ar").

MIND POWER. Visualize bright golden or white light flowing and dissipating from the area of the tumor.

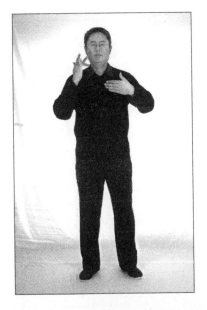

Overactive Thyroid Gland
(hyperthyroidism)

BODY POWER. Near Hand: point middle finger at the thyroid gland; Far Hand: right atrium of the heart (the upper left quadrant of the heart in a frontal view)

SOUL POWER. *Dear soul, mind, and body of my thyroid, I love you. You have the power to heal yourselves. Dear soul, mind, and body of my hands, yi-ar, and light, I love you all. You have the power to heal me. Do a good job. Thank you. Thank you. Thank you.*

SOUND POWER. Chant *yi-ar* (one-two, pronounced "ee-ar").

MIND POWER. Visualize bright golden or white light flowing from the thyroid gland to the right atrium of the heart.

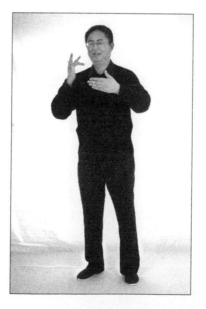

CONDITIONS OF THE LUNGS

Bronchitis, Tracheitis, Pulmonary Emphysema

BODY POWER. Near Hand: affected lung; Far Hand: opposite lung

SOUL POWER. *Dear soul, mind, and body of my lungs, I love you. You have the power to heal yourselves. Dear soul, mind, and body of my hands,* san, *and light, I love you all. You have the power to heal me. Do a good job. Thank you. Thank you. Thank you.*

SOUND POWER. Chant *san* (three, pronounced "sahn").

MIND POWER. Visualize the lungs as completely clear with bright golden or white light dissipating from the affected lung.

Notes

Alternate hands if both lungs are affected.

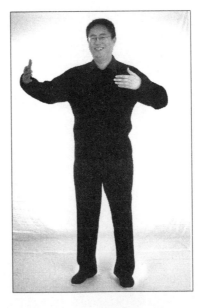

Asthma

Step 1 of 2

BODY POWER. Near Hand: lungs; Far Hand: lower back (Snow Mountain Area)

SOUL POWER. *Dear soul, mind, and body of my lungs, I love you. You have the power to heal yourselves. Dear soul, mind, and body of my hands,* san-jiu, *and light, I love you all. You have the power to heal me. Do a good job. Thank you. Thank you. Thank you.*

SOUND POWER. Chant *san-jiu* (three-nine, pronounced "sahn-joe").

MIND POWER. Visualize bright golden or white light flowing from the lungs to the Snow Mountain Area.

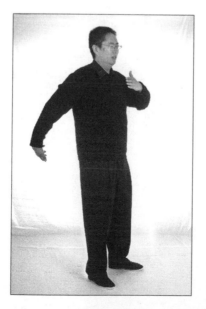

Asthma

Step 2 of 2

BODY POWER. Near Hand: lower back (Snow Mountain Area); Far Hand: lungs

SOUL POWER. *Dear soul, mind, and body of my lungs, I love you. You have the power to heal yourselves. Dear soul, mind, and body of my hands,* jiu-san, *and light, I love you all. You have the power to heal me. Do a good job. Thank you. Thank you. Thank you.*

SOUND POWER. Chant *jiu-san* (nine-three, pronounced "joe-sahn").

MIND POWER. Visualize bright golden or white light flowing from the Snow Mountain Area to the lungs. Visualize the lungs as completely clear and healthy.

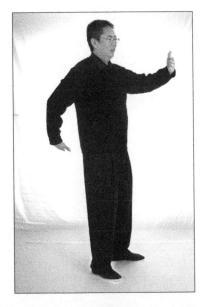

Tuberculosis

Step 1 of 2

BODY POWER. Near Hand: kidney area; Far Hand: lower back (Snow Mountain Area)

SOUL POWER. *Dear soul, mind, and body of my lungs and kidneys, I love you. You have the power to heal yourselves. Dear soul, mind, and body of my hands, jiu, and light, I love you all. You have the power to heal me. Do a good job. Thank you. Thank you. Thank you.*

SOUND POWER. Chant *jiu* (nine, pronounced "joe").

MIND POWER. Visualize bright golden or white light glowing in both kidneys.

Notes

Tuberculosis is typically due to exhaustion of yin energy. The Step 1 procedure builds energy in the kidney area.

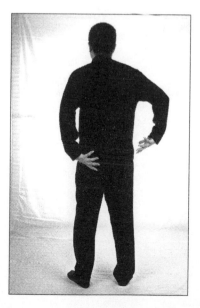

Tuberculosis

Step 2 of 2

BODY POWER. Near Hand: lungs; Far Hand: side of the body

SOUL POWER. *Dear soul, mind, and body of my lungs, I love you. You have the power to heal yourselves. Dear soul, mind, and body of my hands,* san, *and light, I love you all. You have the power to heal me. Do a good job. Thank you. Thank you. Thank you.*

SOUND POWER. Chant *san* (three, pronounced "sahn").

MIND POWER. Visualize the lungs as completely clear and healthy. Visualize bright golden or white light dissipating from the lungs.

Notes

Alternate hands.

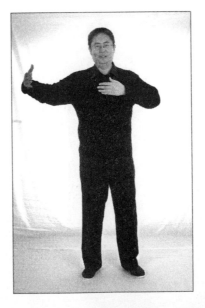

Excess Phlegm

BODY POWER. Near Hand: center of the chest; Far Hand: side of the chest

SOUL POWER. *Dear soul, mind, and body of my lungs, I love you. You have the power to heal yourselves. Dear soul, mind, and body of my hands,* san, *and light, I love you all. You have the power to heal me. Do a good job. Thank you. Thank you. Thank you.*

SOUND POWER. Chant *san* (three, pronounced "sahn").

MIND POWER. Visualize the lungs as completely clear and healthy, with bright golden or white light dissipating from the chest.

Notes

Excess phlegm is due to excess lung energy.

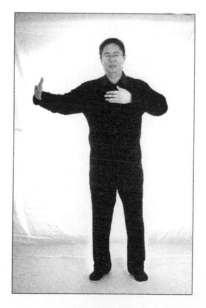

Whooping Cough

(pertussis)

BODY POWER. Near Hand: stomach; Far Hand: lower abdomen (side)

SOUL POWER. *Dear soul, mind, and body of my stomach and chest, I love you. You have the power to heal yourselves. Dear soul, mind, and body of my hands, wu-jiu, and light, I love you all. You have the power to heal me. Do a good job. Thank you. Thank you. Thank you.*

SOUND POWER. Chant *wu-jiu* (five-nine, pronounced "woo-joe").

MIND POWER. Visualize bright golden or white light flowing from the stomach to the lower abdomen.

Notes

In Western medicine, all coughs are thought to be related to the lungs. In traditional Chinese medicine, whooping cough is a "stomach cough," caused by cold air being stuck in the stomach.

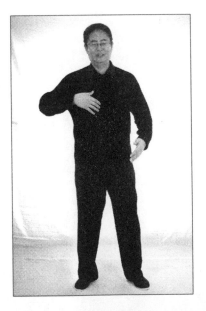

Pneumonia

BODY POWER. Near Hand: lung; Far Hand: lower abdomen (Lower Dan Tian)

SOUL POWER. *Dear soul, mind, and body of my lungs, I love you. You have the power to heal yourselves. Dear soul, mind, and body of my hands,* san-jiu, *and light, I love you all. You have the power to heal me. Do a good job. Thank you. Thank you. Thank you.*

SOUND POWER. Chant *san-jiu* (three-nine, pronounced "sahn-joe").

MIND POWER. Visualize your lungs as completely clear, healthy, and glowing with bright golden or white light.

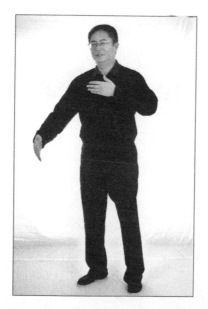

COLDS

Cold

(with lungs clear)

BODY POWER. Near Hand: center of the upper chest; Far Hand: lungs, above nipple level

SOUL POWER. *Dear soul, mind, and body of my chest and lungs, I love you. You have the power to heal yourselves. Dear soul, mind, and body of my hands,* san-wu-jiu, *and light, I love you all. You have the power to heal me. Do a good job. Thank you. Thank you. Thank you.*

SOUND POWER. Chant *san-wu-jiu* (three-five-nine, pronounced "sahn-woo-joe").

MIND POWER. Visualize bright golden or white light dissipating from the chest.

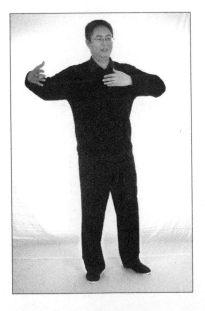

Cold

(with high fever)

BODY POWER. Near Hand: center of the upper chest; Far Hand: extend straight out with the fingers pointing away from the body, above the level of the nipples

SOUL POWER. *Dear soul, mind, and body of my chest and lungs, I love you. You have the power to heal yourselves. Dear soul, mind, and body of my hands,* san-wu, *and light, I love you all. You have the power to heal me. Do a good job. Thank you. Thank you. Thank you.*

SOUND POWER. Chant *san-wu* (three-five, pronounced "sahn-woo").

MIND POWER. Visualize bright golden or white light radiating and dissipating from the chest.

Notes

Follow this procedure for only two minutes, since energy is being directed away from the body with the Far Hand.

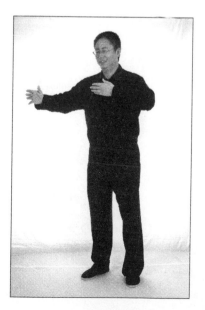

Cold

(after blood loss)

BODY POWER. Near Hand: lower abdomen (Lower Dan Tian); Far Hand: lungs or center of the chest, above nipple level

SOUL POWER. *Dear soul, mind, and body of my chest and lungs, I love you. You have the power to heal yourselves. Dear soul, mind, and body of my hands, jiu-san, and light, I love you all. You have the power to heal me. Do a good job. Thank you. Thank you. Thank you.*

SOUND POWER. Chant *jiu-san* (nine-three, pronounced "joe-sahn").

MIND POWER. Visualize bright golden or white light flowing from the lower abdomen to the lungs.

Notes

Use this procedure when you catch a cold after suffering blood loss from surgery or injury.

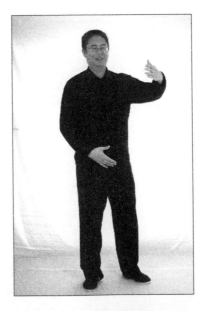

CONDITIONS OF THE HEART

Irregular Heartbeat

(arrhythmia)

BODY POWER. Near Hand: lower abdomen (Lower Dan Tian); Far Hand: slightly below the heart

SOUL POWER. *Dear soul, mind, and body of my heart, I love you. You have the power to heal yourselves. Dear soul, mind, and body of my hands,* jiu-san, *and light, I love you all. You have the power to heal me. Do a good job. Thank you. Thank you. Thank you.*

SOUND POWER. Chant *jiu-san* (nine-three, pronounced "joe-sahn").

MIND POWER. Visualize your heart as healthy. Visualize it glowing with bright golden or white light.

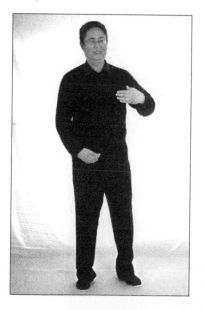

All Other Heart Conditions

BODY POWER. Near Hand: left hand faces left ventricle (left-hand side of heart, to the left of and slightly below left nipple); Far Hand: right hand faces right atrium (right-hand side of heart, to the right of the left nipple and a little higher than the Near Hand)

SOUL POWER. *Dear soul, mind, and body of my heart, I love you. You have the power to heal yourselves. Dear soul, mind, and body of my hands, ar, and light, I love you all. You have the power to heal me. Do a good job. Thank you. Thank you. Thank you.*

SOUND POWER. Chant *ar* (two, pronounced "ar").

MIND POWER. Visualize your heart as healthy. Visualize it glowing with bright golden, white, or red light.

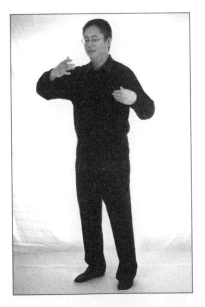

CONDITIONS OF THE SPLEEN AND STOMACH

Stomach Inflammation or Gastritis

Step 1 of 3

BODY POWER. Near Hand: left hand faces the stomach; Far Hand: right hand faces the liver

SOUL POWER. *Dear soul, mind, and body of my stomach and liver, I love you. You have the power to heal yourselves. Dear soul, mind, and body of my hands,* wu-chi, *and light, I love you all. You have the power to heal me. Do a good job. Thank you. Thank you. Thank you.*

SOUND POWER. Chant *wu-chi* (five-seven, pronounced "woo-chi").

MIND POWER. Visualize bright golden or white light flowing from the stomach to the liver.

Notes

After following the Step 1 procedure for two minutes, continue with Step 2. This procedure facilitates portal vein drainage.

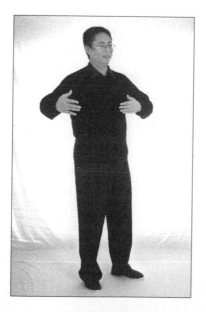

Stomach Inflammation or Gastritis

Step 2 of 3

BODY POWER. Near Hand: point the right hand at the liver and shake it; Far Hand: right atrium of the heart (on the right-hand side of the left nipple)

SOUL POWER. *Dear soul, mind, and body of my stomach, liver, and heart, I love you. You have the power to heal yourselves. Dear soul, mind, and body of my hands, chi-ar, and light, I love you all. You have the power to heal me. Do a good job. Thank you. Thank you. Thank you.*

SOUND POWER. Chant *chi-ar* (seven-two, pronounced "chee-ar").

MIND POWER. Visualize bright golden or white light flowing from the liver to the right auricle.

Notes

Stop after two minutes. Repeat Step 1 and Step 2 for another two minutes each, then end with Step 3.

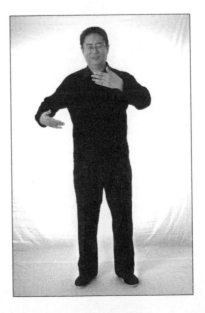

Stomach Inflammation or Gastritis

Step 3 of 3

Body Power. Near Hand: left hand faces left side of the heart, at nipple level (left-hand side of the left nipple); Far Hand: right hand faces right side of the heart, a little higher than the left hand

Soul Power. *Dear soul, mind, and body of my stomach, my heart, and my circulatory system, I love you. You have the power to heal yourselves. Dear soul, mind, and body of my hands,* ar, *and light, I love you all. You have the power to heal me. Do a good job. Thank you. Thank you. Thank you.*

Sound Power. Chant *ar* (two, pronounced "ar").

Mind Power. Visualize your heart as healthy and glowing with bright red light.

Notes

Follow the Step 3 procedure for five minutes. This step promotes blood flow in the whole body.

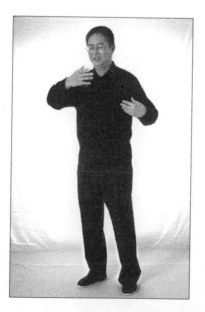

Duodenal Ulcer

BODY POWER. Near Hand: stomach; Far Hand: lower abdomen (Lower Dan Tian)

SOUL POWER. *Dear soul, mind, and body of my stomach ulcer, I love you. You have the power to heal yourselves. Dear soul, mind, and body of my hands,* wu-jiu, *and light, I love you all. You have the power to heal me. Do a good job. Thank you. Thank you. Thank you.*

SOUND POWER. Chant *wu-jiu* (five-nine, pronounced "woo-joe").

MIND POWER. Visualize bright golden or white light dissipating from the stomach area.

Notes

Do this procedure for at most three minutes. Practicing too long may cause descended stomach.

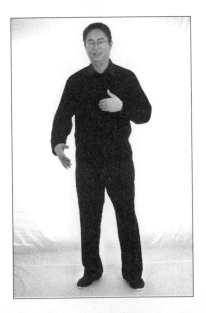

Descended Stomach

BODY POWER. Near Hand: below the stomach; angle the palm slightly upward; Far Hand: upper abdomen

SOUL POWER. *Dear soul, mind, and body of my stomach, I love you. You have the power to heal yourselves. Dear soul, mind, and body of my hands,* jiu-wu, *and light, I love you all. You have the power to heal me. Do a good job. Thank you. Thank you. Thank you.*

SOUND POWER. Chant *jiu-wu* (nine-five, pronounced "joe-woo").

MIND POWER. Visualize the stomach as raised, with bright golden or white light shining in the stomach area.

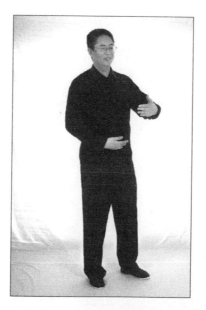

Enlarged Spleen
(splenomegaly)

Step 1 of 3

BODY POWER. Near Hand: left hand faces spleen; Far Hand: right hand faces liver

SOUL POWER. *Dear soul, mind, and body of my spleen, I love you. You have the power to heal yourselves. Dear soul, mind, and body of my hands, chi, and light, I love you all. You have the power to heal me. Do a good job. Thank you. Thank you. Thank you.*

SOUND POWER. Chant *chi* (seven, pronounced "chee").

MIND POWER. Visualize bright golden or white light flowing from the spleen to the liver.

Notes

Do Step 1 for only two to three minutes. Then proceed to Step 2.

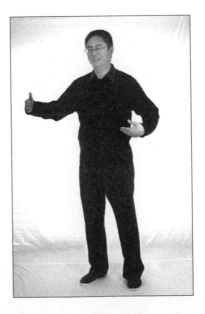

Enlarged Spleen

(splenomegaly)

Step 2 of 3

BODY POWER. Near Hand: liver; Far Hand: center of the chest, above the nipple level

SOUL POWER. *Dear soul, mind, and body of my spleen, I love you. You have the power to heal yourselves. Dear soul, mind, and body of my hands,* chi-ar, *and light, I love you all. You have the power to heal me. Do a good job. Thank you. Thank you. Thank you.*

SOUND POWER. Chant *chi-ar* (seven-two, pronounced "chee-ar").

MIND POWER. Visualize bright golden or white light flowing from the liver to the right atrium (the upper right-hand quadrant of the heart).

Notes

Do Step 2 for only two to three minutes. Proceed with Step 3.

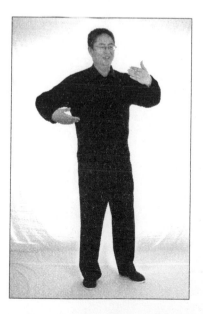

Enlarged Spleen

(splenomegaly)

Step 3 of 3

BODY POWER. Near Hand: left hand faces left side of the heart, at nipple level (left-hand side of the left nipple); Far Hand: right hand faces right side of the heart, a little higher than the left hand

SOUL POWER. *Dear soul, mind, and body of my spleen, my heart, and my circulatory system, I love you. You have the power to heal yourselves. Dear soul, mind, and body of my hands, ar, and light, I love you all. You have the power to heal me. Do a good job. Thank you. Thank you. Thank you.*

SOUND POWER. Chant *ar* (two, pronounced "ar").

MIND POWER. Visualize your heart as healthy and glowing with bright red light.

Notes

Follow the Step 3 procedure for five minutes. This step promotes blood flow in the whole body.

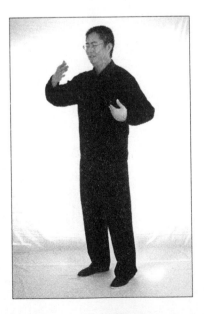

Diabetes

(high blood sugar)

BODY POWER. Near Hand: pancreas or one inch above pancreas (left front stomach area); Far Hand: lower abdomen (Lower Dan Tian); angle the palm slightly upward toward the bladder

SOUL POWER. *Dear soul, mind, and body of my pancreas, I love you. You have the power to heal yourselves. Dear soul, mind, and body of my hands,* wu-jiu, *and light, I love you all. You have the power to heal me. Do a good job. Thank you. Thank you. Thank you.*

SOUND POWER. Chant *wu-jiu* (five-nine, pronounced "woo-joe").

MIND POWER. Visualize bright golden or white light flowing from the pancreas to the lower abdomen.

Notes

Follow this procedure for only three minutes. With diabetes, there is excess energy in the pancreas, and the pancreas does not produce enough insulin. Symptoms and effects usually include excessive thirst and urination. Diabetes takes time to self-heal.

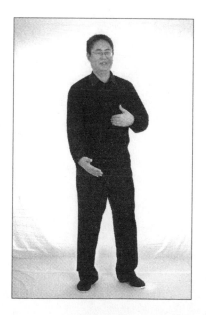

Low Blood Sugar
(hypoglycemia)

BODY POWER. Near Hand: lower abdomen (Lower Dan Tian); Far Hand: pancreas

SOUL POWER. *Dear soul, mind, and body of my pancreas, I love you. You have the power to heal yourselves. Dear soul, mind, and body of my hands, jiu, and light, I love you all. You have the power to heal me. Do a good job. Thank you. Thank you. Thank you.*

SOUND POWER. Chant *jiu* (nine, pronounced "joe").

MIND POWER. Visualize bright golden or white light flowing from the lower abdomen to the pancreas.

Notes

Low blood sugar indicates not enough energy in the pancreas.

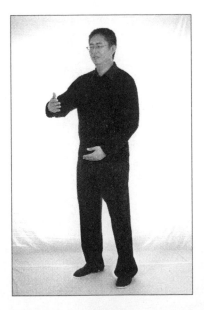

Poor Digestion

BODY POWER. Near Hand: stomach; Far Hand: lower abdomen (Lower Dan Tian)

SOUL POWER. *Dear soul, mind, and body of my stomach, small intestine, and entire digestive system, I love you. You have the power to heal yourselves. Dear soul, mind, and body of my hands,* wu-jiu, *and light, I love you all. You have the power to heal me. Do a good job. Thank you. Thank you. Thank you.*

SOUND POWER. Chant *wu-jiu* (five-nine, pronounced "woo-joe").

MIND POWER. Visualize bright golden or white light flowing from the stomach to the lower abdomen.

Notes

An alternative method is to point one hand to the stomach and chant *San San Jiu Liu Ba Yao Wu* (3396815, pronounced "sahn sahn joe lew bah yow woo").

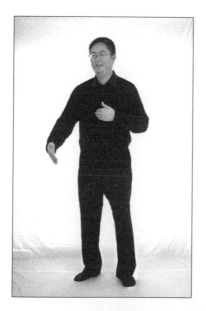

Food Allergies

BODY POWER. Near Hand: stomach; Far Hand: lower abdomen (Lower Dan Tian)

SOUL POWER. *Dear soul, mind, and body of my stomach and my immune system, I love you. You have the power to heal yourselves. Dear soul, mind, and body of my hands,* wu-jiu, *and light, I love you all. You have the power to heal me. Do a good job. Thank you. Thank you. Thank you.*

SOUND POWER. Chant *wu-jiu* (five-nine, pronounced "woo-joe").

MIND POWER. Visualize bright golden or white light flowing from the stomach to the lower abdomen.

Notes

Food allergies indicate too much energy in the stomach area.

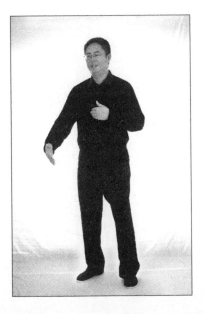

CONDITIONS OF THE LIVER AND GALLBLADDER

Liver Inflammation

BODY POWER. Near Hand: palm faces the liver or the fingers point toward the liver; Far Hand: lower abdomen (Lower Dan Tian)

SOUL POWER. *Dear soul, mind, and body of my liver, I love you. You have the power to heal yourselves. Dear soul, mind, and body of my hands,* chi-jiu, *and light, I love you all. You have the power to heal me. Do a good job. Thank you. Thank you. Thank you.*

SOUND POWER. Chant *chi-jiu* (seven-nine, pronounced "chee-joe").

MIND POWER. Visualize bright golden or white light flowing from the liver to the lower abdomen.

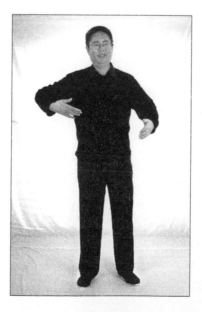

Enlarged Liver

Step 1 of 3

BODY POWER. Near Hand: left hand faces the stomach; Far Hand: right hand faces the liver

SOUL POWER. *Dear soul, mind, and body of my stomach and liver, I love you. You have the power to heal yourselves. Dear soul, mind, and body of my hands,* wu-chi, *and light, I love you all. You have the power to heal me. Do a good job. Thank you. Thank you. Thank you.*

SOUND POWER. Chant *wu-chi* (five-seven, pronounced "woo-chee").

MIND POWER. Visualize bright golden or white light flowing from the stomach to the liver.

Notes

After following the Step 1 procedure for two minutes, continue with Step 2. These procedures facilitate portal vein drainage.

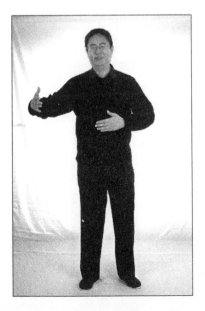

Enlarged Liver

Step 2 of 3

BODY POWER. Near Hand: liver; Far Hand: center of the chest (Message Center)

SOUL POWER. *Dear soul, mind, and body of my liver and heart, I love you. You have the power to heal yourselves. Dear soul, mind, and body of my hands,* chi-ar, *and light, I love you all. You have the power to heal me. Do a good job. Thank you. Thank you. Thank you.*

SOUND POWER. Chant *chi-ar* (seven-two, pronounced "chee-ar").

MIND POWER. Visualize bright golden or white light flowing from the liver to the right atrium of the heart (on the right-hand side of the left nipple).

Notes

Stop after two minutes. Repeat Steps 1 and 2 for another two minutes each. Then end with Step 3.

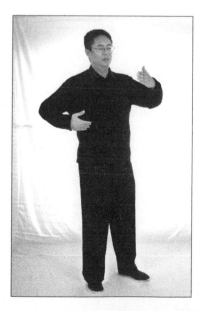

Enlarged Liver

Step 3 of 3

BODY POWER. Near Hand: left hand faces left side of the heart, at nipple level (left-hand side of the left nipple); Far Hand: right hand faces right side of the heart, a little higher than the left hand

SOUL POWER. *Dear soul, mind, and body of my liver, my heart, and my circulatory system, I love you. You have the power to heal yourselves. Dear soul, mind, and body of my hands,* ar, *and light, I love you all. You have the power to heal me. Do a good job. Thank you. Thank you. Thank you.*

SOUND POWER. Chant *ar* (two, pronounced "ar").

MIND POWER. Visualize your heart as healthy and glowing with bright red light.

Notes

Follow the Step 3 procedure for five minutes. This step promotes blood flow in the whole body.

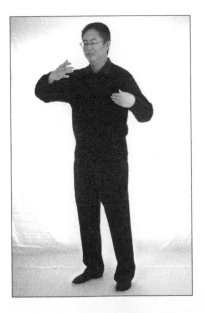

Jaundice

(caused by hepatitis)

BODY POWER. Near Hand: liver; Far Hand: bladder area; pointing slightly downward

SOUL POWER. *Dear soul, mind, and body of my liver, I love you. You have the power to heal yourselves. Dear soul, mind, and body of my hands, chi-jiu, and light, I love you all. You have the power to heal me. Do a good job. Thank you. Thank you. Thank you.*

SOUND POWER. Chant *chi-jiu* (seven-nine, pronounced "chee-joe").

MIND POWER. Visualize bright golden or white light flowing from the liver to the lower abdomen.

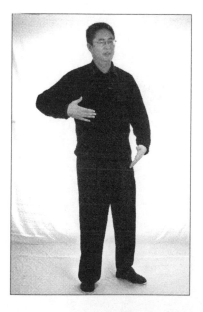

Cirrhosis of the Liver

Step 1 of 3

BODY POWER. Near Hand: lower abdomen (Lower Dan Tian); Far Hand: liver

SOUL POWER. *Dear soul, mind, and body of my liver, I love you. You have the power to heal yourselves. Dear soul, mind, and body of my hands,* jiu-chi, *and light, I love you all. You have the power to heal me. Do a good job. Thank you. Thank you. Thank you.*

SOUND POWER. Chant *jiu-chi* (nine-seven, pronounced "joe-chee").

MIND POWER. Visualize bright golden or white light flowing from the lower abdomen to the liver.

Notes

Follow the procedure in Step 1 for only two to three minutes. Then proceed with Step 2.

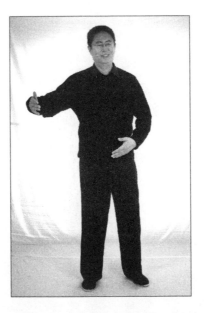

Cirrhosis of the Liver

Step 2 of 3

BODY POWER. Near Hand: liver; Far Hand: center of the chest, above nipple level

SOUL POWER. *Dear soul, mind, and body of my liver, I love you. You have the power to heal yourselves. Dear soul, mind, and body of my hands,* chi-ar, *and light, I love you all. You have the power to heal me. Do a good job. Thank you. Thank you. Thank you.*

SOUND POWER. Chant *chi-ar* (seven-two, pronounced "chee-ar").

MIND POWER. Visualize the liver being raised and bright golden or white light flowing from the liver to the right atrium of the heart.

Notes

Follow the procedure in Step 2 for only two minutes. Then proceed with Step 3.

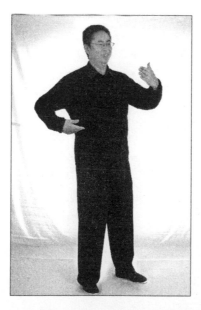

Cirrhosis of the Liver

Step 3 of 3

BODY POWER. Near Hand: left hand faces left side of the heart, at nipple level (left-hand side of the left nipple); Far Hand: right hand faces right side of the heart, a little higher than the left hand

SOUL POWER. *Dear soul, mind, and body of my liver, my heart, and my circulatory system, I love you. You have the power to heal yourselves. Dear soul, mind, and body of my hands, ar, and light, I love you all. You have the power to heal me. Do a good job. Thank you. Thank you. Thank you.*

SOUND POWER. Chant *ar* (two, pronounced "ar").

MIND POWER. Visualize your heart as healthy and glowing with bright red light.

Notes

Practice Step 3 for five minutes. Hardening of the liver tissues is due to inadequate cellular vibration in the liver. Therefore, cirrhosis indicates not enough energy in the liver.

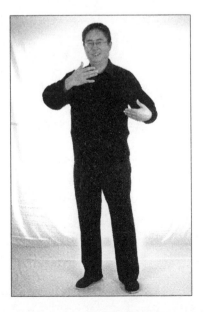

Hepatitis B and C

BODY POWER. Near Hand: liver; shake the Near Hand; Far Hand: lower abdomen (Lower Dan Tian)

SOUL POWER. *Dear soul, mind, and body of my liver, I love you. You have the power to heal yourselves. Dear soul, mind, and body of my hands,* chi-jiu, *and light, I love you all. You have the power to heal me. Do a good job. Thank you. Thank you. Thank you.*

SOUND POWER. Chant *chi-jiu* (seven-nine, pronounced "chee-joe").

MIND POWER. Visualize bright golden or white light radiating and dissipating from the liver.

Notes

Hepatitis B is a condition in which there are too few liver cells, and too much energy in those few cells.

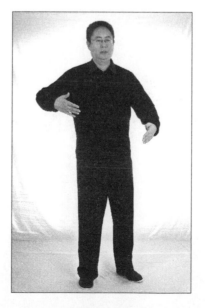

Gallstones and Gallbladder Inflammation
(cholecystitis)

Step 1 of 2

BODY POWER. Near Hand: point middle finger at the gallbladder (right front rib area); Far Hand: lower abdomen (Lower Dan Tian)

SOUL POWER. *Dear soul, mind, and body of my gallbladder, I love you. You have the power to heal yourselves. Dear soul, mind, and body of my hands,* chi-jiu, *and light, I love you all. You have the power to heal me. Do a good job. Thank you. Thank you. Thank you.*

SOUND POWER. Chant *chi-jiu* (seven-nine, pronounced "chee-joe").

MIND POWER. Visualize bright golden or white light flowing from the gallbladder to the lower abdomen.

Notes

When gallstones move out of the gallbladder, you may feel severe pain. Use the procedure in Step 2 at this point.

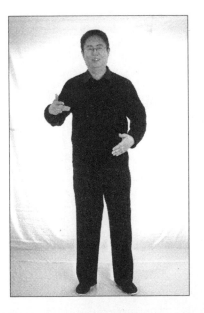

Gallstones and Gallbladder Inflammation

Step 2 of 2

(Use for breaking up gallstones; skip this step for inflammation.)

BODY POWER. Near Hand: lower abdomen (Lower Dan Tian); Far Hand: gallbladder area

SOUL POWER. *Dear soul, mind, and body of my gallbladder, I love you. You have the power to heal yourselves. Dear soul, mind, and body of my hands,* jiu-chi, *and light, I love you all. You have the power to heal me. Do a good job. Thank you. Thank you. Thank you.*

SOUND POWER. Chant *jiu-chi* (nine-seven, pronounced "joe-chee").

MIND POWER. Visualize a laser beam of bright golden or white light breaking up the gallstones.

Notes

Step 2 is used to transfer energy from the Lower Dan Tian to break up the gallstones.

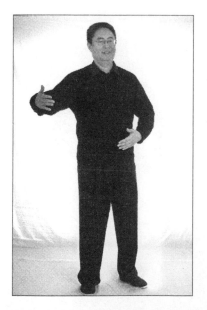

CONDITIONS OF THE KIDNEYS AND BLADDER

Kidney Inflammation, Kidney Atrophy, Kidney Stones

(acute and chronic nephritis)

BODY POWER. Near Hand: affected kidney; Far Hand: other kidney or the lower back (Snow Mountain Area)

SOUL POWER. *Dear soul, mind, and body of my kidneys, I love you. You have the power to heal yourselves. Dear soul, mind, and body of my hands, jiu, and light, I love you all. You have the power to heal me. Do a good job. Thank you. Thank you. Thank you.*

SOUND POWER. Chant *jiu* (nine, pronounced "joe").

MIND POWER. Visualize bright golden or white light dissipating from the kidney area.

Notes

If there is a kidney stone or a tumor, point at it with the middle finger of the Near Hand. Visualize a bright golden or white laser beam of light from the finger to the stone or tumor, dissolving it.

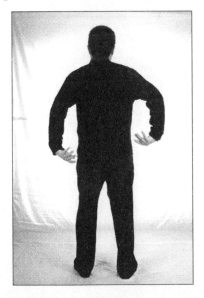

Urinary Tract Inflammation, Bladder Inflammation
(urethritis, cystitis)

Acute Conditions

BODY POWER. Near Hand: bladder area; Far Hand: other side of the bladder; point the fingers down a bit to help dissipate excess energy

SOUL POWER. *Dear soul, mind, and body of my bladder, I love you. You have the power to heal yourselves. Dear soul, mind, and body of my hands, jiu, and light, I love you all. You have the power to heal me. Do a good job. Thank you. Thank you. Thank you.*

SOUND POWER. Chant *jiu* (nine, pronounced "joe").

MIND POWER. Visualize bright golden or white light dissipating from the bladder area.

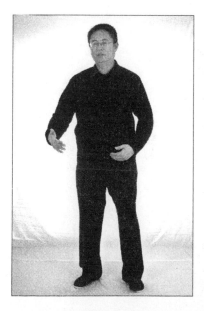

Urinary Tract Inflammation, Bladder Inflammation

Chronic Conditions

Step 1 of 2

BODY POWER. Near Hand: bottom of the bladder at the lower abdomen; Far Hand: side of the bladder (spend three minutes on each side)

SOUL POWER. *Dear soul, mind, and body of my bladder, I love you. You have the power to heal yourselves. Dear soul, mind, and body of my hands,* jiu, *and light, I love you all. You have the power to heal me. Do a good job. Thank you. Thank you. Thank you.*

SOUND POWER. Chant *jiu* (nine, pronounced "joe").

MIND POWER. Visualize bright golden or white light radiating from the bladder.

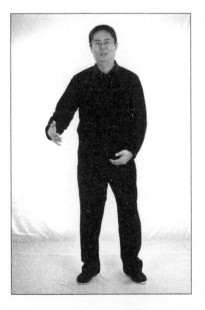

Urinary Tract Inflammation, Bladder Inflammation

Chronic Conditions

Step 2 of 2

BODY POWER. Near Hand: bladder; Far Hand: lower abdomen (Lower Dan Tian)

SOUL POWER. *Dear soul, mind, and body of my bladder, I love you. You have the power to heal yourselves. Dear soul, mind, and body of my hands,* jiu, *and light, I love you all. You have the power to heal me. Do a good job. Thank you. Thank you. Thank you.*

SOUND POWER. Chant *jiu* (nine, pronounced "joe").

MIND POWER. Visualize bright golden or white light dissipating from the bladder area.

Notes

Constricted blood vessels in the wall of the bladder and the urinary tract result in not enough blood flow and not enough energy in the tissues.

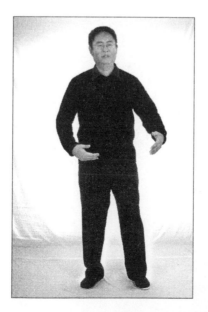

Polyps or Tumors in the Bladder

BODY POWER. Near Hand: point the middle finger at the polyp or tumor in the bladder; Far Hand: lower abdomen (side)

SOUL POWER. *Dear soul, mind, and body of my tumors and bladder, I love you. You have the power to heal yourselves. Dear tumors, you've gone in the wrong direction. Turn back to normal cells. You can do it. Dear soul, mind, and body of my hands,* jiu, *and light, I love you all. You have the power to heal me. Do a good job. Thank you. Thank you. Thank you.*

SOUND POWER. Chant *jiu* (nine, pronounced "joe").

MIND POWER. Visualize bright golden or white light dissipating from the bladder.

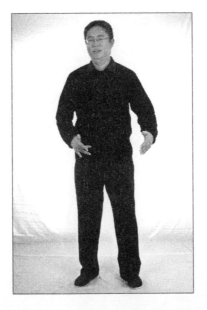

CONDITIONS OF THE LOWER ABDOMEN

Enlarged or Inflamed Prostate

BODY POWER. Near Hand: point the middle finger at the prostate, and shake or wiggle it; Far Hand: lower abdomen (side)

SOUL POWER. *Dear soul, mind, and body of my prostate, I love you. You have the power to heal yourselves. Dear soul, mind, and body of my hands,* jiu, *and light, I love you all. You have the power to heal me. Do a good job. Thank you. Thank you. Thank you.*

SOUND POWER. Chant *jiu* (nine, pronounced "joe").

MIND POWER. Visualize bright golden or white light dissipating from the prostate gland. Imagine the prostate shrinking and returning to normal size.

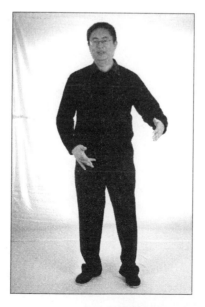

Pain Around the Navel

BODY POWER. Near Hand: point the middle finger at the painful area; Far Hand: another part of the abdomen

SOUL POWER. *Dear soul, mind, and body of my navel, I love you. You have the power to heal yourselves. Dear soul, mind, and body of my hands,* jiu, *and light, I love you all. You have the power to heal me. Do a good job. Thank you. Thank you. Thank you.*

SOUND POWER. Chant *jiu* (nine, pronounced "joe").

MIND POWER. Visualize bright golden or white light dissipating from the navel area.

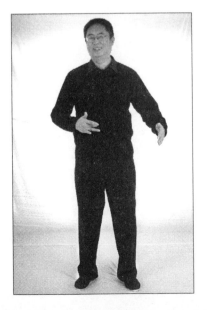

Diarrhea

BODY POWER. Near Hand: lower abdomen (Lower Dan Tian); Far Hand: stomach or upper abdomen

SOUL POWER. *Dear soul, mind, and body of my digestive system, I love you. You have the power to heal yourselves. Dear soul, mind, and body of my hands, jiu-wu, and light, I love you all. You have the power to heal me. Do a good job. Thank you. Thank you. Thank you.*

SOUND POWER. Chant *jiu-wu* (nine-five, pronounced "joe-woo").

MIND POWER. Visualize bright golden or white light flowing from the lower abdomen to the stomach.

Notes

Diarrhea is caused by lack of cellular vibration in the digestive organs. Increase fluid intake to maintain electrolyte balance and to prevent dehydration if the condition persists. For chronic diarrhea, try eating a bulb of roasted garlic daily for a few days.

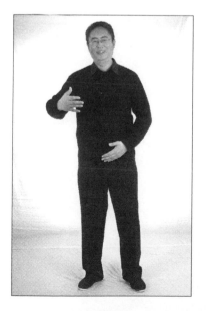

Constipation

BODY POWER. Near Hand: upper abdomen; Far Hand: lower abdomen (side)

SOUL POWER. *Dear soul, mind, and body of my large intestine and lungs, I love you. You have the power to heal yourselves. Dear soul, mind, and body of my hands,* wu-jiu, *and light, I love you all. You have the power to heal me. Do a good job. Thank you. Thank you. Thank you.*

SOUND POWER. Chant *wu-jiu* (five-nine, pronounced "woo-joe").

MIND POWER. Visualize bright golden or white light flowing from the upper abdomen to the lower abdomen.

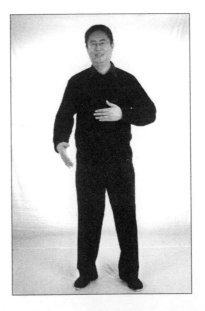

Incontinence

BODY POWER. Near Hand: Zhong Jie acupuncture point, four *cun* (roughly 4 inches) below the navel; Far Hand: lower back (Snow Mountain Area)

SOUL POWER. *Dear soul, mind, and body of my bladder and urinary tract, I love you. You have the power to heal yourselves. Dear soul, mind, and body of my hands, jiu, and light, I love you all. You have the power to heal me. Do a good job. Thank you. Thank you. Thank you.*

SOUND POWER. Chant *jiu* (nine, pronounced "joe").

MIND POWER. Visualize bright golden or white light flowing from the Snow Mountain Area to the bladder and urinary tract.

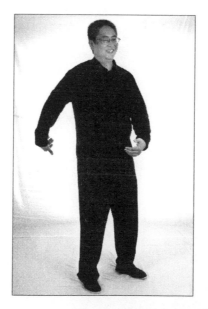

Hemorrhoids

BODY POWER. Near Hand: anus area; Far Hand: lower abdomen (Lower Dan Tian)

SOUL POWER. *Dear soul, mind, and body of my anus or hemorrhoid area, I love you. You have the power to heal yourselves. You have too much energy; send your excess energy to the Lower Dan Tian. Dear soul, mind, and body of my hands,* shi-jiu, *and light, I love you all. You have the power to heal me. Do a good job. Thank you. Thank you. Thank you.*

SOUND POWER. Chant *shi-jiu* (ten-nine, pronounced "shih-joe").

MIND POWER. Visualize a bright golden or white beam of light flowing from the hemorrhoid area to the Lower Dan Tian.

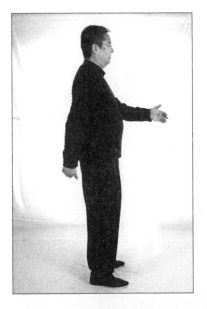

FEMININE CONDITIONS

Uterine Fibroids

BODY POWER. Near Hand: point the middle finger at the area of the fibroid(s) or tumor(s); Far Hand: side of the lower abdomen

SOUL POWER. *Dear soul, mind, and body of my uterus, I love you. You have the power to heal yourselves. Dear soul, mind, and body of my hands, jiu, and light, I love you all. You have the power to heal me. Do a good job. Thank you. Thank you. Thank you.*

SOUND POWER. Chant *jiu* (nine, pronounced "joe").

MIND POWER. Visualize bright golden or white light dissipating from the uterus.

Notes

Blood clots will form (a good sign) when the tumor begins dissipating. If uterine bleeding resumes (discharge changes from a brown color to a red color), stop this practice and use the following healing procedure.

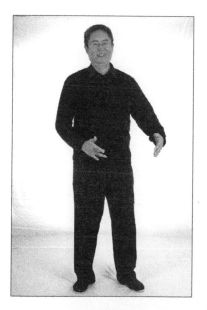

277

Heavy Periods (menorrhagia)
or Bleeding from Uterine Fibroids

BODY POWER. Near Hand: uterus, palm facing slightly upward; Far Hand: upper abdomen, palm angled slightly downward

SOUL POWER. *Dear soul, mind, and body of my uterus, I love you. You have the power to heal yourselves. Dear soul, mind, and body of my hands,* jiu-wu, *and light, I love you all. You have the power to heal me. Do a good job. Thank you. Thank you. Thank you.*

SOUND POWER. Chant *jiu-wu* (nine-five, pronounced "joe-woo").

MIND POWER. Visualize bright golden or white light flowing from the uterus to the upper abdomen.

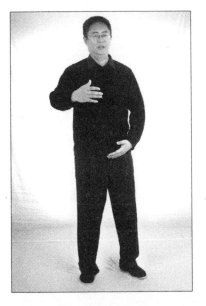

Breast Lumps, Cysts, and Tumors

BODY POWER. Near Hand: point the middle finger at the area of the cyst; Far Hand: other breast

SOUL POWER. *Dear soul, mind, and body of my breast(s), I love you. You have the power to heal yourselves. Dear soul, mind, and body of my hands,* san *(or* ar*), and light, I love you all. You have the power to heal me. Do a good job. Thank you. Thank you. Thank you.*

SOUND POWER. Chant *san* or *ar* (three, pronounced "sahn," or two, pronounced "ar").

MIND POWER. Visualize bright golden or white light radiating from the cyst area.

Notes

Alternate hands if there are cysts in both breasts.

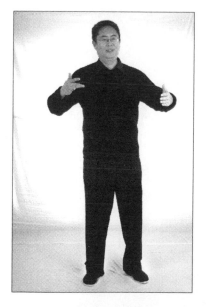

CONDITIONS OF THE BLOOD VESSELS

Temperature Imbalance in the Body

BODY POWER. Near Hand: warm side of the body, at the chest or lung; Far Hand: opposite side (the cold side of the body)

SOUL POWER. *Dear soul, mind, and body of my heart and circulatory system, I love you. You have the power to heal yourselves. Dear soul, mind, and body of my hands, ar, and light, I love you all. You have the power to heal me. Do a good job. Thank you. Thank you. Thank you.*

SOUND POWER. Chant *ar* (two, pronounced "ar").

MIND POWER. Visualize bright golden or white light radiating from the warm part of the body to the cold part.

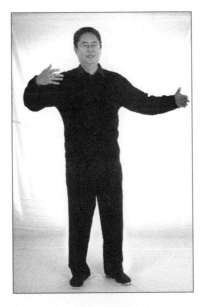

Inflammation of the Aorta

(arteritis)

BODY POWER. Near Hand: center of the chest (Message Center); Far Hand: with the hand at chest level, extend the fingers straight out

SOUL POWER. *Dear soul, mind, and body of my heart, I love you. You have the power to heal yourselves. Dear soul, mind, and body of my hands,* ar, *and light, I love you all. You have the power to heal me. Do a good job. Thank you. Thank you. Thank you.*

SOUND POWER. Chant *ar* (two, pronounced "ar").

MIND POWER. Visualize bright golden or white light dissipating from the heart area.

Notes

This is an emergency situation! Call 911 first. Then follow this procedure for at most three minutes.

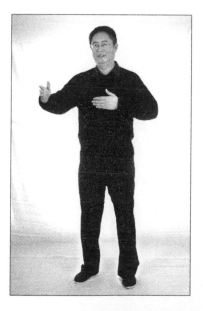

Inflammation of the Veins
(phlebitis)

BODY POWER. Near Hand: point four fingers up the affected leg at the site of the inflamed veins; Far Hand: right atrium of the heart, above nipple level

SOUL POWER. *Dear soul, mind, and body of my heart, I love you. You have the power to heal yourselves. Dear soul, mind, and body of my hands,* shiyi-ar, *and light, I love you all. You have the power to heal me. Do a good job. Thank you. Thank you. Thank you.*

SOUND POWER. Chant *shiyi-ar* (eleven-two, pronounced "shih-ee-ar").

MIND POWER. Visualize bright golden or white light flowing from the affected veins to the right atrium of the heart.

Notes

If there is a heavy feeling or swelling in the legs after standing or walking, work on improving circulation.

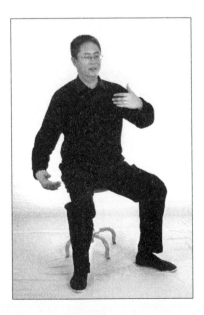

CONDITIONS OF THE BONES AND JOINTS

Neck Pain

(caused by wind)

BODY POWER. Near Hand: back of neck; Far Hand: lower abdomen (Lower Dan Tian)

SOUL POWER. *Dear soul, mind, and body of my neck, I love you. You have the power to heal yourselves. Dear soul, mind, and body of my hands,* yi-jiu, *and light, I love you all. You have the power to heal me. Do a good job. Thank you. Thank you. Thank you.*

SOUND POWER. Chant *yi-jiu* (one-nine, pronounced "ee-joe").

MIND POWER. Visualize bright golden or white light flowing from the neck to the lower abdomen.

Notes

Unprotected exposure to too much wind (natural energy) can lead to an accumulation and blockage of energy in the body, causing pain and stiffness.

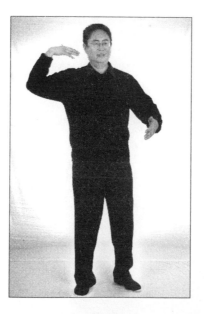

Cervical Bone Spur

BODY POWER. Near Hand: point the middle finger at the affected area at the back of the neck; Far Hand: lower abdomen (Lower Dan Tian)

SOUL POWER. *Dear soul, mind, and body of my neck, I love you. You have the power to heal yourselves. Dear soul, mind, and body of my hands,* yi-jiu, *and light, I love you all. You have the power to heal me. Do a good job. Thank you. Thank you. Thank you.*

SOUND POWER. Chant *yi-jiu* (one-nine, pronounced "ee-joe").

MIND POWER. Visualize bright golden or white light dissipating from the area of the spur.

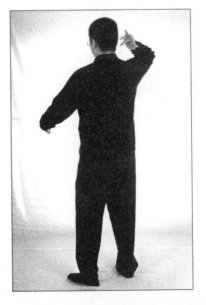

Frozen Shoulder

BODY POWER. Near Hand: affected shoulder; Far Hand: lower abdomen (Lower Dan Tian)

SOUL POWER. *Dear soul, mind, and body of my shoulder, I love you. You have the power to heal yourselves. Dear soul, mind, and body of my hands,* shiyi-jiu, *and light, I love you all. You have the power to heal me. Do a good job. Thank you. Thank you. Thank you.*

SOUND POWER. Chant *shiyi-jiu* (eleven-nine, pronounced "shih-ee-joe").

MIND POWER. Visualize bright golden or white light flowing from the affected shoulder to the chest.

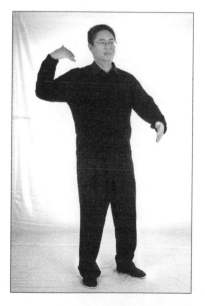

Adhesions in Shoulders

(muscles and tendons stuck together)

BODY POWER. Near Hand: over affected shoulder, shaking; Far Hand: lower abdomen (Lower Dan Tian)

SOUL POWER. *Dear soul, mind, and body of my shoulder, I love you. You have the power to heal yourselves. Dear soul, mind, and body of my hands,* shiyi-jiu, *and light, I love you all. You have the power to heal me. Do a good job. Thank you. Thank you. Thank you.*

SOUND POWER. Chant *shiyi-jiu* (eleven-nine, pronounced "shih-ee-joe").

MIND POWER. Visualize bright golden or white light dissipating in the affected area.

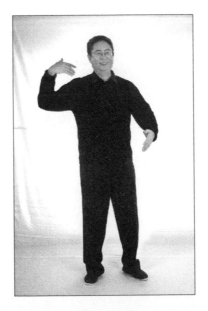

Lower Back Problems

(osteoarthritis, lumbar spine)

BODY POWER. Near Hand: point the middle finger upward at the affected area; Far Hand: ribs

SOUL POWER. *Dear soul, mind, and body of my lower back, I love you. You have the power to heal yourselves. Dear soul, mind, and body of my hands,* jiu-liu, *and light, I love you all. You have the power to heal me. Do a good job. Thank you. Thank you. Thank you.*

SOUND POWER. Chant *jiu-liu* (nine-six, pronounced "joe-lew").

MIND POWER. Visualize bright golden or white light dissipating in the affected area.

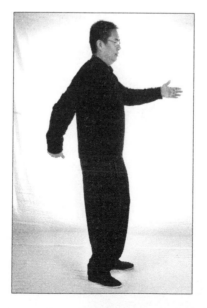

Slipped Disc

(herniated lumbar disc)

BODY POWER. Near Hand: lower abdomen (Lower Dan Tian); Far Hand: lower back, facing the area of the slipped disc

SOUL POWER. *Dear soul, mind, and body of my slipped disc and spinal column, I love you. You have the power to heal yourselves. Dear soul, mind, and body of my hands, jiu, and light, I love you all. You have the power to heal me. Do a good job. Thank you. Thank you. Thank you.*

SOUND POWER. Chant *jiu* (nine, pronounced "joe").

MIND POWER. Visualize bright golden or white light flowing from the lower abdomen to the affected area.

Notes

This condition is a result of weak back energy (weak Du meridian), unless caused by trauma or sports injury.

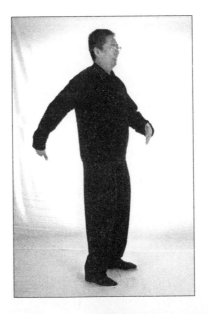

Pain in the Lower Back and Down the Leg
(sciatica)

BODY POWER. Near Hand: palm faces the affected area; alternatively, point the middle finger at the area; Far Hand: lower abdomen (Lower Dan Tian) or other side of the body, at hip level

SOUL POWER. *Dear soul, mind, and body of my back, legs, and nerves, I love you. You have the power to heal yourselves. Dear soul, mind, and body of my hands,* shiyi-jiu, *and light, I love you all. You have the power to heal me. Do a good job. Thank you. Thank you. Thank you.*

SOUND POWER. Chant *shiyi-jiu* (eleven-nine, pronounced "shih-ee-joe).

MIND POWER. Visualize bright golden or white light flowing from the affected area to the lower abdomen or to the other side of the body.

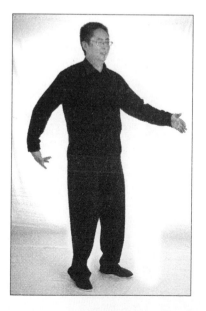

Lower Back Pain

BODY POWER. Near Hand: painful side of the back; Far Hand: opposite side of the back

SOUL POWER. *Dear soul, mind, and body of my back, I love you. You have the power to heal yourselves. Dear soul, mind, and body of my hands,* jiu, *and light, I love you all. You have the power to heal me. Do a good job. Thank you. Thank you. Thank you.*

SOUND POWER. Chant *jiu* (nine, pronounced "joe").

MIND POWER. Visualize bright golden or white light dissipating from the painful side of the back.

Notes

Alternate the hands.

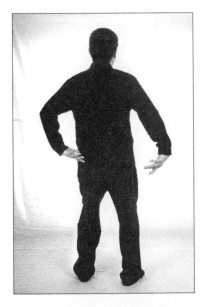

Arthritic Pain in the Knee

(osteoarthritis of the knee)

BODY POWER. Near Hand: affected knee; Far Hand: other knee

SOUL POWER. *Dear soul, mind, and body of my knees, I love you. You have the power to heal yourselves. Dear soul, mind, and body of my hands,* shiyi, *and light, I love you all. You have the power to heal me. Do a good job. Thank you. Thank you. Thank you.*

SOUND POWER. Chant *shiyi* (eleven, pronounced "shih-ee").

MIND POWER. Visualize bright golden or white light dissipating in the painful area of the affected knee.

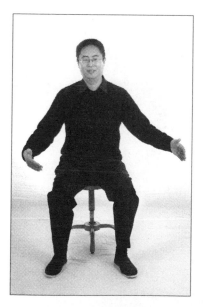

Ankle Pain

BODY POWER. Using the One-Hand Healing technique, point all four fingers at the affected area.

SOUL POWER. *Dear soul, mind, and body of my ankle, I love you. You have the power to heal yourselves. Dear soul, mind, and body of my hands,* shiyi, *and light, I love you all. You have the power to heal me. Do a good job. Thank you. Thank you. Thank you.*

SOUND POWER. Chant *shiyi* (eleven, pronounced "shih-ee").

MIND POWER. Visualize bright golden or white light dissipating from the ankle.

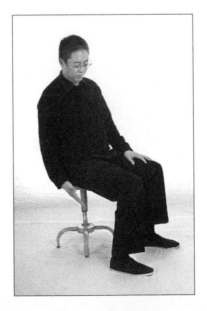

Inflammation of the Bone Marrow

(osteomyelitis)

BODY POWER. Near Hand: over the affected bone; Far Hand: lower part of the affected area

SOUL POWER. *Dear soul, mind, and body of my bones, I love you. You have the power to heal yourselves. Dear soul, mind, and body of my hands,* shiyi, *and light, I love you all. You have the power to heal me. Do a good job. Thank you. Thank you. Thank you.*

SOUND POWER. Chant *shiyi* (eleven, pronounced "shih-ee").

MIND POWER. Visualize bright golden or white light flowing downward from the affected area.

Notes

This procedure directs energy downward from the affected area; otherwise the infection could spread through the bone marrow.

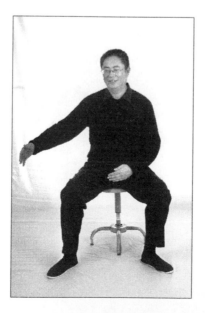

Cavities in the Bone Marrow
(osteomyelitic cavitation)

BODY POWER. Near Hand: lower abdomen (Lower Dan Tian); Far Hand: affected area

SOUL POWER. *Dear soul, mind, and body of my bones, I love you. You have the power to heal yourselves. Dear soul, mind, and body of my hands,* jiu, *and light, I love you all. You have the power to heal me. Do a good job. Thank you. Thank you. Thank you.*

SOUND POWER. Chant *jiu* (nine, pronounced "joe"); if the affected area is a limb, use *jiu-shiyi* (nine-eleven, pronounced "joe-shih-ee").

MIND POWER. Visualize bright golden or white light flowing from the lower abdomen to the affected area.

Notes

This procedure directs energy downward from the affected area; otherwise the infection could spread through the bone marrow.

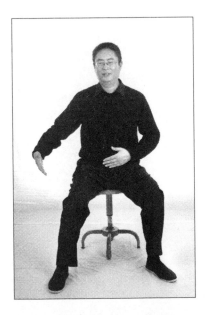

Low Bone Density

(osteoporosis)

BODY POWER. Near Hand: lower abdomen (Lower Dan Tian); Far Hand: affected area

SOUL POWER. *Dear soul, mind, and body of my bones, I love you. You have the power to heal yourselves. Dear soul, mind, and body of my hands, jiu, and light, I love you all. You have the power to heal me. Do a good job. Thank you. Thank you. Thank you.*

SOUND POWER. Chant *jiu* or *jiu-shiyi* (nine, pronounced "joe," or nine-eleven, pronounced "joe-shih-ee").

MIND POWER. Visualize your bones, your entire skeleton as strong, dense, full of energy, and glowing brightly with golden or white light.

Notes

Think of the Snow Mountain Area strengthening and building the energy of the kidneys. The Snow Mountain Area provides energy food for the kidneys, which in turn are related to the bones.

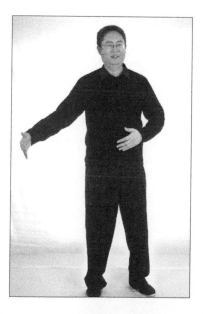

CONDITIONS OF THE SKIN

Burn

(new)

BODY POWER. Near Hand: area of the burn; Far Hand: lower abdomen (Lower Dan Tian)

SOUL POWER. *Dear soul, mind, and body of my skin, I love you. You have the power to heal yourselves. Dear soul, mind, and body of my hands, jiu, and light, I love you all. You have the power to heal me. Do a good job. Thank you. Thank you. Thank you.*

SOUND POWER. Chant *x-jiu* (x-nine, pronounced x-"joe"). The first healing number depends on the location of the burn. Refer to table 7 on page 179. For example, if the burn is on your face, use *yi-jiu* (one-nine, pronounced "ee-joe").

MIND POWER. Visualize bright golden or white light flowing from the area of the burn to the lower abdomen.

Notes

New burns are areas where the tissues have too much energy. This procedure transfers the excess energy to the Lower Dan Tian, the body's storehouse of energy.

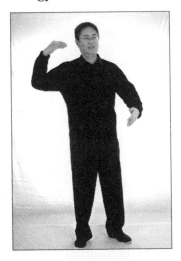

Burn

(old)

BODY POWER. Near Hand: lower abdomen (Lower Dan Tian); Far Hand: area of the burn

SOUL POWER. *Dear soul, mind, and body of my burn, I love you. You have the power to heal yourselves. Turn back to normal skin. You can do it. Dear soul, mind, and body of my hands,* jiu, *and light, I love you all. You have the power to heal me. Do a good job. Thank you. Thank you. Thank you.*

SOUND POWER. Chant *jiu-x* (nine-x, pronounced "joe"-x). The second healing number depends on the location of the burn. Refer to table 7 on page 179. For example, if the burn is on your face, use *jiu-yi* (nine-one, pronounced "joe-ee").

MIND POWER. Visualize bright golden or white light flowing from the lower abdomen to the burn area.

Notes

Old burns recover slowly due to insufficient energy in the burn area. This procedure sends energy from the Lower Dan Tian to the area of the old burn.

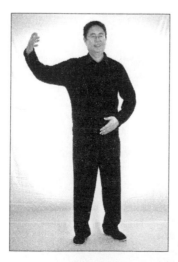

Psoriasis

(of the head)

BODY POWER. Near Hand: affected side of the head; Far Hand: other side of the head

SOUL POWER. *Dear soul, mind, and body of my head and skin, I love you. You have the power to heal yourselves. Dear soul, mind, and body of my hands, yi, and light, I love you all. You have the power to heal me. Do a good job. Thank you. Thank you. Thank you.*

SOUND POWER. Chant *yi* (one, pronounced "ee").

MIND POWER. Visualize bright golden or white laser light removing the affected skin.

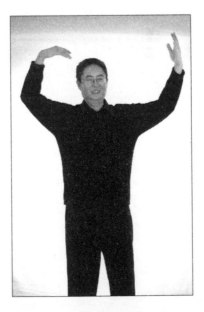

Athlete's Foot

BODY POWER. Using the One-Hand Healing technique, point all four fingers at the affected foot. Angle the fingers slightly upward.

SOUL POWER. *Dear soul, mind, and body of my feet, I love you. You have the power to heal yourselves. Dear soul, mind, and body of my hand,* shiyi, *and light, I love you all. You have the power to heal me. Do a good job. Thank you. Thank you. Thank you.*

SOUND POWER. Chant *shiyi* (eleven, pronounced "shih-ee").

MIND POWER. Visualize bright golden or white light dissipating from the affected area, leaving the skin of the feet glowing and healthy.

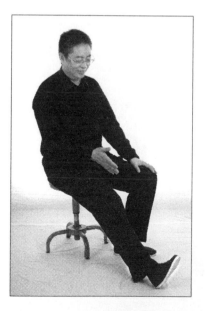

Acne and Facial Blemishes

BODY POWER. Near Hand: point the middle finger at the blemish or pimple; Far Hand: any other part of the face

SOUL POWER. *Dear soul, mind, and body of my face, you have the power to heal yourselves. Dear soul, mind, and body of my hands,* yi, *and light, I love you all. You have the power to heal me. Do a good job. Thank you. Thank you. Thank you.*

SOUND POWER. Chant *yi* (one, pronounced "ee").

MIND POWER. Visualize bright golden or white light dissipating from the blemish or pimple.

Notes

Alternate the hands if both sides of the face are affected.

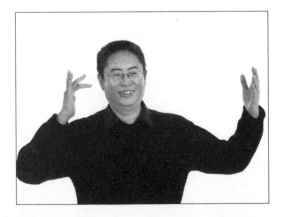

Preventive Maintenance

You've now seen the breadth, depth — and simplicity — of the theory and application of Soul Mind Body Medicine for healing. In chapter 7, I gave you a healing handbook, a "user's manual" of Soul Mind Body Medicine for more than one hundred of the most common physical ailments. But Soul Mind Body Medicine has still more to offer you. Five thousand years ago, the *Yellow Emperor's Canon*, the authoritative text of traditional Chinese medicine, stated: *The best doctor is one who teaches people how to prevent sickness, not one who treats sickness.* What was true then is true now. I believe that in the future medicine will increasingly focus on prevention of illness rather than on treating and healing it once it has manifested. If you are healthy, Soul Mind Body Medicine can help you maintain good health. In this chapter we will explore how.

KEY FACTORS IN PREVENTING ILLNESS

As you have learned, the key factors in healing are the removal of blockages (energy, matter, and spiritual) and balance — in the transformation between matter and energy at the cellular level, in the flow of energy throughout the body, and in soul, mind, and body. Balance and the removal of blockages are vital for prevention of illness as well. This includes balance in your daily schedule, your emotions, and your diet. Next, you need to develop your body's five most important energy centers. Finally, I will show you four simple daily practices to promote these keys to preventing illness. Combined, these practices take less than twenty-five minutes to do. First let's examine some key factors in healing.

Daily Regularity

Go to sleep early, wake up early, and eat your meals on time. This is such simple wisdom, but it is so important in preventing illness. Maintain your biological rhythms in a regular, smooth, and harmonized way. Adhering to a regular daily schedule is vital for maintaining good energy, vitality, and immunity to prevent illness.

Stress Management

People may have different levels of stress and different levels of tolerance for stress, but stress is absolutely inimical to health. When you are stressed, your immune system function declines, your endocrine system, nervous system, cardiovascular system, digestive system — all your body systems — can become unbalanced. Here is one very simple and effective practice to reduce stress:

According to Soul Mind Body Medicine, stress is an energy blockage in the head. Removing the energy blockage in the head will reduce your stress right away. Apply the Four Power Techniques:

BODY POWER. Sit in a chair. Keep your back straight, and don't lean back against the chair. Use the One Hand Near, One Hand Far Body Power technique. Point your Near Hand at the crown chakra at the top of your head. This hand should be held about four to seven inches above your head. Place your Far Hand fifteen to twenty inches away from your lower abdomen, with the palm facing your body. The Near Hand creates a high-density field at the head, while the Far Hand creates a low-density field at the lower abdomen. Energy will flow from high density (the head) to low density (the lower abdomen), dissipating the energy blockage in the head and reducing stress. At the same time, your foundational energy centers will be nourished and strengthened.

SOUL POWER. Say "hello": *Dear soul, mind, and body of my head, lower abdomen, Near Hand, Far Hand, ee-joe (one-nine), and the brightest golden light, I love you. Please give me a healing to reduce my stress. Do a good job. Thank you.*

The combined Soul Power of your head, abdomen, and hands, combined with *ee-joe* and the brightest golden light, can offer incredible healing to reduce your stress.

SOUND POWER. Chant the healing sounds of the numbers one and nine in Chinese, pronounced "ee" and "joe," respectively. *Ee* stimulates cellular vibration in the head. *Joe* stimulates cellular vibration in the lower abdomen. Chanting *ee-joe* repeatedly will move blocked energy from the head to the lower abdomen, reducing your stress.

MIND POWER. Visualize the brightest golden light flowing from the head to the lower abdomen. The intention of your mind, coupled with the vibration of the cells in your brain and head, will move blocked energy from the head to the lower abdomen. Visualize or imagine yourself in perfect health and being completely calm and relaxed, full of inner joy and peace.

Do this practice for three to five minutes. Repeat it several times a day as needed. You can use it to prevent stress as well as to reduce it.

Diet

A great deal of good guidance is available on this subject from dieticians. Here are a few simple dietary guidelines:

Eat Less

Try eating less, especially if you are concerned about excess weight. Gradually reduce your food intake until you are eating 70 to 80 percent of what you are eating now. Try not to eat to the point of being totally full at any meal. Eating until you are full increases the burden on your digestive system.

Eat More Vegetables, Fruit, and Proper Protein

The following guidance for simple food intake is very important for general health and prevention of illness. If you eat enough vegetables and fruits, you will get enough vitamins and minerals. If you are deficient in vitamins or minerals, as determined by testing, you can take supplements. By following these guidelines, you can take care of your daily protein and calcium requirements. Every day, eat:

- one egg
- a little meat (chicken, fish, pork, beef)
- one glass of milk or two glasses of soy milk for calcium

Drink at least eight glasses of water a day. After eating, take a slow five-to-ten-minute walk, which will greatly aid digestion and absorption.

Developing the Body's Energy Centers

Our five most important energy centers are the Lower Dan Tian, the Snow Mountain Area, the Message Center or Middle Dan Tian, the Zu Qiao, and the Third Eye or Upper Dan Tian (see figure 26, p. 306). Developing the power of these five energy centers is key to preventing illness, maintaining good health, and prolonging life.

Lower Dan Tian

LOCATION

The Lower Dan Tian is located 1.5 *cun* (about one inch) below the navel and 2.5 *cun* inside your body. It is roughly the size of your fist.

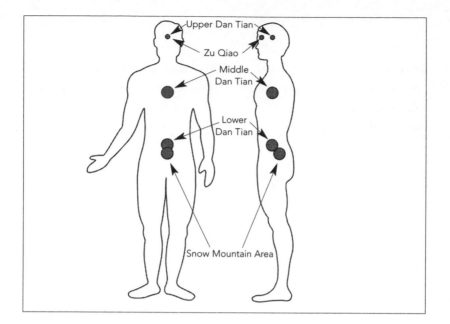

Figure 26.

The five most important energy centers

SIGNIFICANCE

The Lower Dan Tian is:

- a foundational energy center

- key to stamina, vitality, and immunity

- key to long life

- the postnatal energy center

- the seat of the soul

DEVELOPING THE LOWER DAN TIAN

Apply the Four Power Techniques to develop the power of the Lower Dan Tian:

BODY POWER. Grip your left thumb with your right palm, using 80 percent of your maximum strength. Close both palms. Place this

Yin/Yang Palm (see figure 1, p. 43) on your lower abdomen, in front of your Lower Dan Tian.

SOUL POWER. Say "hello": *Dear soul, mind, and body of my Lower Dan Tian, I love you. Please boost your own energy. Do a good job. Thank you.*

SOUND POWER. Chant *jiu* (pronounced "joe"), the number nine in Chinese.

MIND POWER. Visualize the brightest golden light from the universe pouring into your Lower Dan Tian to form a powerful, bright, concentrated light ball there.

Figure 27 shows the practice in a basic seated position. Figure 29 shows the practice in an advanced, full-lotus position. In the advanced position you can build power more rapidly. An intermediate alternative is shown in figure 28. With feet shoulder-width apart and knees slightly bent, hold both hands near (four to seven inches away from) the Lower Dan Tian on either side, as shown. The Soul Power, Sound Power, and Mind Power techniques remain the same, whatever your body posture.

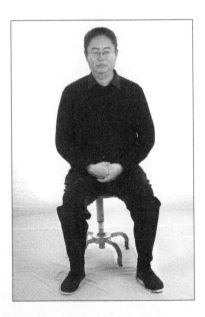

Figure 27.

Develop Lower Dan Tian (seated)

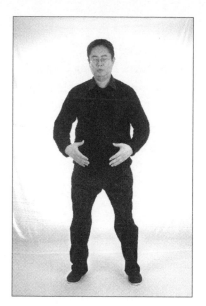

Figure 28.

Develop Lower Dan Tian (standing)

For preventive maintenance, do this exercise in any of these positions for three to five minutes each day. If you want to build a strong, healthy body and prolong your life, or to build your immunity and vitality, do this exercise for a half hour or even longer each day. The Lower Dan Tian is essential to your foundational power.

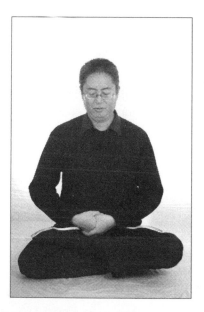

Figure 29.

Develop Lower Dan Tian (full lotus)

Snow Mountain Area

LOCATION

Imagine a straight line connecting your navel to your back. Divide this line into three equal parts. Go inside your back to the end of the first segment (in other words, go one-third of the way inside your body, starting from your back). From this point, go down 2.5 *cun.* This is the center of the Snow Mountain Area, which is roughly the size of your fist.

SIGNIFICANCE

The Snow Mountain Area is:

- the prenatal energy center, which connects with the energy of your parents and your ancestors and holds the essence of their energy
- key to quality of life and long life
- the energy source for the kidneys
- energy food for the brain and Third Eye
- the starting point of four major meridians (Ren, Du, Dai, and Chong; see chapter 6)

Snow Mountain Area is a Buddhist term. Taoists call this area the Golden Urn. Traditional Chinese medicine calls it the Ming Men Area, which means the "gate of life." In yoga, this area is the kundalini. Developing the power of the Snow Mountain Area is vital.

DEVELOPING THE SNOW MOUNTAIN AREA

Apply the Four Power Techniques to develop the power of the Snow Mountain Area:

BODY POWER. Hold your hands behind your back with the palms facing the kidneys. Hold the Near Hand four to seven inches away from one kidney, and the Far Hand fifteen to twenty inches away from the other kidney (see figure 31, p. 309). Alternate your Near and

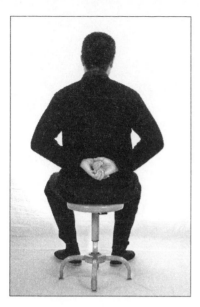

Figure 30.

Develop Snow Mountain Area (seated)

Far Hands, since they will tire. You may also place the Yin/Yang Palm over your Snow Mountain Area, as shown in figures 30 and 32 (p. 310).

SOUL POWER. Say "hello": *Dear soul, mind, and body of my Snow Mountain Area, the sun, my Near Hand, and Far Hand, I love you*

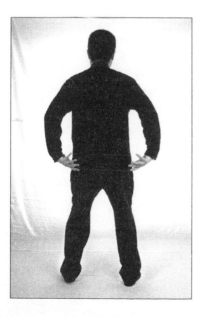

Figure 31.

Develop Snow Mountain Area (standing)

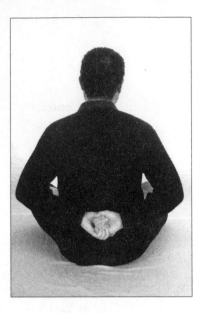

Figure 32.

Develop Snow Mountain Area (full lotus)

all. You have the power to develop the power of my Snow Mountain Area. Do a good job. Thank you. Thank you. Thank you.

SOUND POWER. Chant *sunlight, sunlight, sunlight, sunlight.*

MIND POWER. Visualize a mountain of snow in your Snow Mountain Area, with the sun shining down from above. The warmth of the sun is melting the snow. As the snow melts and turns to water, steam rises and nourishes your entire body.

For preventive maintenance, do this exercise for three to five minutes each day. If you want to build a strong, healthy body and prolong your life, or build a strong foundation for opening your Third Eye, do this exercise for a half hour or even longer each day. You will receive many benefits.

Message Center (Middle Dan Tian)

LOCATION

From the point in the middle of your chest between the nipples, go 2.5 *cun* inside the body. This is the center of the Message Center or Middle Dan Tian, which is roughly the size of your fist. The Message Center is also known as the heart chakra.

SIGNIFICANCE

The Message Center is one of the most important energy centers because it is the center for:

- *Soul communication.* After opening the Message Center, you can converse directly with the Divine and the universe.

- *Soul Language.* After developing the Message Center, you can speak and translate Soul Language and use Soul Language to heal, bless, and receive guidance from the Divine and the universe.

- *Healing.* The Message Center is the repository of your strongest healing powers.

- *Emotions.* Balancing and developing the Message Center can correct any emotional imbalances.

- *Love, forgiveness, and compassion.* Through the Message Center, you can offer love, forgiveness, and compassion to yourself and to others. Love melts any blockage. Forgiveness brings peace and inner joy. Compassion gives you strength. Love and forgiveness are the keys to healing and to advancing on your spiritual journey.

- *Life transformation.* All aspects of your life connect with your Message Center. Clearing the energy and spiritual blockages in the Message Center can transform your life instantly.

- *Karma.* The Message Center stores your karma (the mistakes you have made in all your lifetimes). Clear your karma, and healing, blessing, and life transformation will follow instantly.

- *Soul enlightenment.* On the spiritual journey, enlightening your soul is one of the highest goals. To reach soul enlightenment, you must purify your soul, mind, and body; cleanse your spiritual blockages; and fully commit to offering universal service, including universal love, forgiveness, peace, healing, blessing, harmony, and enlightenment.

DEVELOPING THE MESSAGE CENTER

Apply the Four Power Techniques to develop the power of the Message Center:

BODY POWER. Bring your hands together in front of your chest. Leave your right hand in this "prayer" position, but drop your left hand to cover your Message Center (or heart chakra) in the middle of your chest, without touching, as illustrated in figures 33, 34, and 35. This hand position helps open your Message Center.

SOUL POWER. Say "hello": *Dear soul, mind, and body of my Message Center, I love you. You are the healing, life transformation, and soul enlightenment center. Please open yourself. You can do it. Do a good job. Thank you. Dear soul, mind, and body of my hands, of* San San Jiu Liu Ba Yao Wu (3396815), *and of Sha's Golden Healing Ball, I*

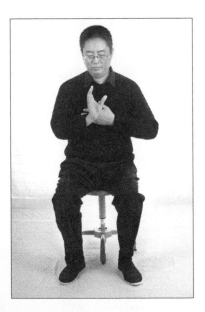

Figure 33.

Develop Message Center (seated)

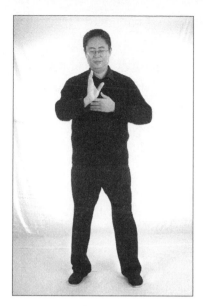

Figure 34.

Develop your Message Center (standing)

love you. Please give an extraordinary blessing to my Message Center to open it fully. I am very honored and appreciative. Thank you. Thank you. Thank you. Dear San San Jiu Liu Ba Yao Wu, *dear Sha's Golden Healing Ball, please come from Heaven to rotate counterclockwise rapidly in my Message Center.*

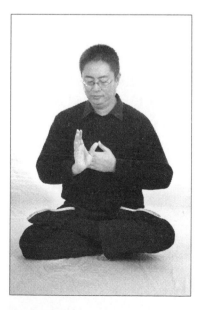

Figure 35.

Develop your Message Center (full lotus)

SOUND POWER. Chant 3396815 in Chinese (pronounced "sahn sahn joe lew bah yow woo") as fast as you can.

MIND POWER. Visualize Sha's Golden Healing Ball spinning quickly in the Message Center to clear and purify the Message Center.

For preventive maintenance, do this exercise for three to five minutes each day. Practice more for more benefits, or practice the following special meditation:

MEDITATION FOR OPENING THE MESSAGE CENTER

The power of the Message Center is unlimited. Even after it is opened, it can always be opened further. Because it is the key center for healing the soul, mind, and body and for both physical life and the spiritual journey, let me lead you in a powerful meditation to clear and open your Message Center.

Sit on the floor in the full- or half-lotus position, or with your legs crossed naturally. You may also sit in a chair. Be comfortable, but keep your back straight, and do not lean back against the chair. Place the tip of your tongue close to, but not touching, the roof of your mouth. Contract your anus slightly. Close your eyes and relax. Hold both hands in front of your Message Center with the heels of your palms, your thumbs, and your pinkies touching gently. Open the other fingers wide, like a lotus flower.

Chant *San San Jiu Liu Ba Yao Wu, San San Jiu Liu Ba Yao Wu, San San Jiu Liu Ba Yao Wu, San San Jiu Liu Ba Yao Wu* as fast as you can. At the same time, rotate Sha's Golden Healing Ball counterclockwise as quickly as you can in your Message Center. So far, this is identical to the basic exercise for developing the Message Center described above.

Now ask Sha's Golden Healing Ball to expand. Step-by-step, Sha's Golden Healing Ball becomes as large as your room, your home, your block, your neighborhood, your city, your state, your country, your continent, your hemisphere, Mother Earth, the solar system, the galaxy, the universe — and beyond.

The secret to this meditation is that as you visualize Sha's Golden

Healing Ball expanding within your Message Center, your Message Center and you yourself are expanding with it. When Sha's Golden Healing Ball expands to the size of Mother Earth, your Message Center is the size of Mother Earth also. When Sha's Golden Healing Ball expands to the size of the universe, your Message Center is the universe. The universe is one, the Divine is one, and *you* are one with the universe. All the light from the universe pours into your Message Center to open, purify, nourish, transform, and enlighten your Message Center.

Next, reverse the process. Contract the ball — and your Message Center — gradually. Bring them back to your physical self. The ball contracts from the size of the universe to the galaxy, the solar system, Mother Earth, your country, your city, your room, back to you. As your Message Center contracts, it retains and concentrates all the light from the universe.

Practice this special meditation for at least seven minutes, the longer the better. The more often you practice this meditation, the better, since it can open your Message Center very quickly.

Zu Qiao

LOCATION

The Zu Qiao (pronounced "zoo chow") is located inside the bone cavity behind the Yin Tang acupuncture point, which is between your eyebrows. It is roughly the size of a cherry.

SIGNIFICANCE

The Zu Qiao is the key center for Mind Power, the potential power of the brain. As we know, we each have about 15 billion brain cells, but in our entire life, we typically use only 10 to 15 percent of them. The 85 to 90 percent of brain cells that we do not use remain dormant. I call them potential cells. Developing the potential cells of the brain is one of our major tasks of the twenty-first century. The Zu Qiao is the energy center that directly supports the development of the potential power of the brain.

DEVELOPING THE ZU QIAO

Apply the Four Power Techniques to develop the power of the Zu Qiao:

BODY POWER. Face the palm of your Near Hand to the Yin Tang acupuncture point between your eyebrows. Hold the palm of your Far Hand a few inches in front of the Near Hand (see figures 36, 37, 38). Alternate hands if you get tired. The energy generated by your palms in this secret Body Power position will radiate to and stimulate cellular vibration in the Zu Qiao. The resulting energy from the Zu Qiao will in turn radiate back to the palms. In this way, energy radiates back and forth between the palms and the Zu Qiao, with a constant stimulating and reinforcing effect.

SOUL POWER. Say "hello": *Dear soul, mind, and body of my Zu Qiao; dear soul, mind, and body of my hands; dear soul, mind, and body of yi,* the number one; *dear soul, mind, and body of universal light, I love you. Please build the power of my Zu Qiao. I am very honored and blessed. Thank you. Thank you. Thank you.*

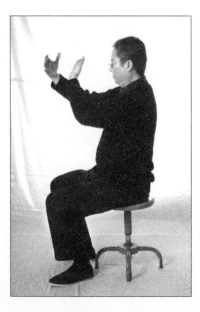

Figure 36.

Develop Zu Qiao (seated)

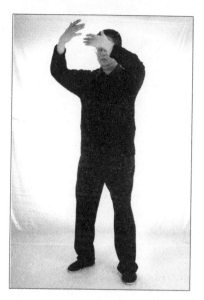

Figure 37.

Develop Zu Qiao
(standing)

SOUND POWER. Chant the number one, *yi*, in Chinese (pronounced "ee"). "Ee" vibrates the entire head and brain, including the Zu Qiao.

MIND POWER. Visualize the brightest light radiating in the Zu Qiao area. Visualize the light pouring into the Zu Qiao area from the entire universe. The light concentrates into a ball. Concentrate

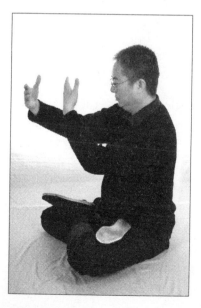

Figure 38.

Develop Zu Qiao
(full lotus)

this light ball further. Condense this light ball. Increase the density of this ball, making it brighter and brighter.

Do this exercise for at least seven minutes each day, the longer, the better.

Third Eye (Upper Dan Tian)

LOCATION

The Third Eye, also known as the Upper Dan Tian, is a cherry-sized energy center located in the center of your head. Specifically, from the midpoint between your eyebrows, draw a line going straight up to the top of your head. Draw another line over your head connecting the tops of both ears. At the point where these two lines cross, go down three *cun* into your head. This is the location of the Third Eye, which corresponds with the location of the pineal gland.

SIGNIFICANCE

The Third Eye is one of the major spiritual centers of the body. When you develop and open the Third Eye, you will be able to see images of the spiritual world, enabling you to glean more wisdom from it. The Third Eye also supports Mind Power, contributing to the development of the brain's potential power.

DEVELOPING THE THIRD EYE

Before you do any Third Eye development, you must develop solid foundational energy centers, particularly the Snow Mountain Area. The Snow Mountain Area is the foundation of the Third Eye because it provides energy food for it. If you try to develop the Third Eye without a proper foundation, you will become tired, weak, even drained. You may also weaken your immune system and experience other health problems. First do the "Developing the Snow Mountain Area" exercise (see p. 308) for at least fifteen minutes — and preferably thirty minutes — every day for a month. If you have headaches, hypertension, glaucoma, a brain tumor, brain cancer, Alzheimer's, or are recovering from a stroke, do *not* practice any Third Eye exercises, because these illnesses involve energy blockages in the brain. Apply the Four Power Techniques to develop and open the Third Eye:

BODY POWER. Use the One Hand Near, One Hand Far healing technique, with both hands above the crown of your head on slightly opposite sides, as shown in figures 39, 40, and 41. The fingertips of both hands will radiate energy to stimulate the Third Eye.

SOUL POWER. Say "hello": *Dear soul, mind, and body of my Third Eye, I love you. Please develop your capabilities to see images of the spiritual world. Dear soul, mind, and body of my hands, of 01777-908, 01777-92244* (see chapter 3, p. 47), *of Sha's Golden Healing Ball, and of all the cities, countries, Mother Earth, all the planets, galaxies, and infinite universes, I love you all. Could you all work together? Expand my Third Eye. Turn my Third Eye into the entire universe to receive blessings from the entire universe. I am honored and blessed. Thank you. Thank you. Thank you.*

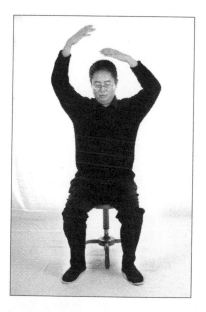

Figure 39.

Develop Third Eye (seated)

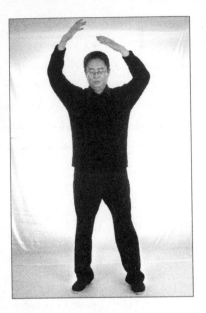

Figure 40.

Develop the Third Eye (standing)

SOUND POWER. We will use 01777-908 and 01777-92244, the codes or mantras described in chapter 3, to develop the potential power of the brain, including the Third Eye. Chant *ling yow chee chee chee, joe ling bah, ling yow chee chee chee, joe ar ar sih sih* (pronunciation in Chinese) throughout this practice.

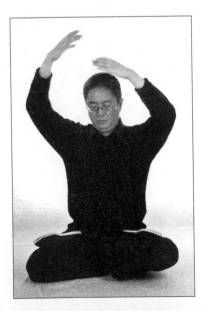

Figure 41.

Develop the Third Eye (full lotus)

MIND POWER. Visualize two Sha's Golden Healing Balls, one flowing out from your right and one from your left fingers. Picture them entering your head and then colliding and merging with your Third Eye. The single merged ball spins counterclockwise, expanding in size and increasing in brightness and intensity. As in the meditation for opening the Message Center (p. 314), expand the ball to the size of your room, home, neighborhood, city, state, country, Mother Earth, the solar system, the galaxy, the universe. Your Third Eye expands with the ball. When the ball expands to the size of the universe, your Third Eye also expands to the size of the universe. The ball *is* the entire universe. Your Third Eye *is* the entire universe. Universal light fills your entire Third Eye. Your Third Eye constantly receives the nourishment of the universe. At the same time, the wisdom of the universe pours into it.

Then contract the size of the ball back from the universe, galaxies, Mother Earth, country, city, your home, and into your physical self. As the ball contracts, the light from the universe, galaxies, planets, Mother Earth, your country, city, and home pours into your Third Eye. The light ball concentrates in your Third Eye. As you condense the ball, as it concentrates and gets smaller and smaller, it also gets brighter and brighter, and it becomes smarter.

Expand and contract Sha's Golden Healing ball and your Third Eye again in the same way. Do it repeatedly. Do this exercise for at least seven minutes, the longer the better. This practice will develop your Third Eye very quickly. Immediately after Third Eye practice, spend five minutes grounding yourself. Place the Yin/Yang Palm (see figure 1, p. 43) on your lower abdomen. Concentrate on your lower abdomen, visualizing a golden light ball spinning there. After about five minutes, your energy will be grounded.

After you practice this exercise you could wind up with a headache or a heavy feeling in the head and brain. The headache could even be severe and would be a sign that your Third Eye is developing. What you are feeling is energy radiating from the strong cellular vibration of your Third Eye. Generally speaking, try to tolerate any pain caused by the vibration of your Third Eye. If you cannot tolerate the pain, use the Four Power Techniques, including One Hand Near, One Hand Far, to release the headache. See chapter 7, pp. 183–86.

On the spiritual journey, many people have a strong desire to open their Third Eye. Remember one of the deepest spiritual principles: Follow nature's way. Do not force anything. Do the proper practice, and do it properly. If your Third Eye opens, say, *Thank you.* If your Third Eye does not respond, also say *Thank you.* It takes some time to open it. Do not rush things. The Third Eye always opens suddenly, often when you are extremely tired.

DAILY PRACTICE

Every day you have to eat food, drink water, and sleep. These are the basic necessities. On top of that, the daily practice of Soul Mind Body Medicine will greatly benefit you.

Below I offer you four daily practices. They are very simple exercises to promote your energy flow, maintain your good health, increase your immunity, help you heal and prevent illness, and balance your soul, mind, and body.

WAKING UP (ONE MINUTE)

Before you get out of bed, say: *Good morning, Divine* [or whatever fits your belief system]. *I thank you very much for all your blessings in my life. Dear soul, mind, and body of 3396815* (pronounced "sahn sahn joe lew bah yow woo"), *dear soul, mind, and body of Sha's Golden Healing Ball, I love you. Could you give me a blessing to promote energy and blood flow throughout my body? Help remove every blockage in my body, increase my immunity, and bless every aspect of my life today. I am very honored and blessed. Thank you. Thank you. Thank you.*

Then chant *San San Jiu Liu Ba Yao Wu* continuously for one minute. At the same time, visualize Sha's Golden Healing Ball coming from the universe to your body, spinning from head to toe and skin to bone. After one minute, say: *Hao. Hao. Hao. Thank you. Thank you. Thank you.*

WENG AR HONG (TEN MINUTES)

Apply the Four Power Techniques:

BODY POWER. Stand with your legs shoulder-width apart. Put your right hand about three inches above your navel, and your left hand about three inches below the navel, both palms facing up (see figure 8, p. 55). If you have hypertension, glaucoma, a brain tumor, or cancer, hold your right palm face down.

SOUL POWER. Say "hello": *Dear soul, mind, and body of every system in my body, every organ, every cell, and every strand of DNA and RNA, could you boost your own energy, vitality, and immunity? You have the power to do it. Do a good job. Thank you. Dear soul, mind, and body of Weng Ar Hong, could you give me a blessing to stimulate cellular vibration throughout my body? I am very honored and blessed. Thank you. Thank you. Thank you.*

SOUND POWER. Inhale deeply. Exhale in one breath and chant *Weng Ar Hong* (pronounced "wung ar hohng"). Chant *Weng Ar Hong* in one breath repeatedly.

MIND POWER. Visualize bright red light in your head when you chant *Weng*. Visualize bright white light in your chest when you chant *Ar*. Visualize bright blue light in your abdomen when you chant *Hong*.

Do this exercise for ten minutes. You can practice Weng Ar Hong anytime during the day, but the best time to practice is in the early morning. Face the sun and practice outdoors if possible. You can receive incredible blessings from the sunlight and fresh air.

UNIVERSAL CONNECTION AND MEDITATION (TEN MINUTES)

Sit down comfortably. Keep your back straight and free of any support. Almost touch both thumbs together, with the fingers of the right hand resting in the palm of the left hand (see figure 3, p. 47). This hand position is called Universal Connection.

Apply Universal Meditation. Visualize anything you wish in your lower abdomen. For example, you can visualize the ocean, with ships floating on the waves and fish swimming; mountains with homes, trees, flowers, and animals; real and imaginary planets; and universes. Put whatever comes into your mind at the moment into your lower abdomen. Allow whatever you visualize to give you love, compassion, and blessings. At the same time, give your love and care to whatever you visualize. You serve them. They serve you. You are applying universal service. When more people on Mother Earth and more souls in the universe follow this practice, world peace and universal harmony will be reached sooner.

Do this exercise for at least ten minutes. If you are fortunate enough to go into a deep meditative state, I suggest that you continue the exercise without regard to time. When you finish the exercise, a few hours may have passed. If you can reach that stage of meditation, you are extremely blessed.

GOING TO SLEEP (ONE MINUTE)

Lie in bed on your back. Place your left palm on your abdomen below the navel, and your right palm above the

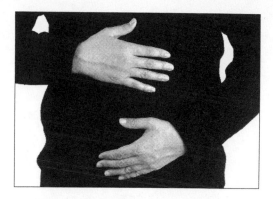

Figure 42.

Building the Foundation

navel (see figure 42, p. 49). This hand position is called Building the Foundation. We will practice a sacred mantra of Guan Yin, the Goddess of Compassion.

SOUL POWER. Say "hello": *Dear soul, mind, and body of Weng Ma Ni Ba Ma Hong, please give me a blessing for total health and peace and enlighten my soul. Thank you. Thank you. Thank you.*

Then chant *Weng Ma Ni Ba Ma Hong* for one minute. At the same time, visualize Ling Hui Sheng Shi (the name given by the Divine to Guan Yin, the Goddess of Compassion) smiling at you and blessing you. You yourself are filled with golden light, with perfect health, and with inner joy and peace. Close this exercise in the usual way, by saying: *Hao. Hao. Hao. Thank you. Thank you. Thank you. Gong song. Gong song. Gong song.*

❧⟨◯⟩☙

Completing these four daily practices takes less than twenty-five minutes. They are vital for boosting your energy, vitality, and stamina and for preventing sickness, maintaining good health, and improving the quality of your life.

Healing is important, but prevention of illness is even more important. Do not wait until you are sick to try to fix things. Maintain your good health with these daily practices for soul, mind, and body.

The Essence

In this book, I have shared my deepest wisdom and knowledge of
Soul Mind Body Medicine. Some of this information has been kept
secret since ancient times. I believe that this knowledge cannot be
hidden anymore; it must be revealed to benefit you and all of humanity. As a universal servant, I have held back nothing. The only way to
receive new wisdom is to share the old. Following this spiritual law
has served me well. It is like emptying a warehouse to make room for
new goods. Without sharing and teaching from my heart, I could not
learn as much, or be given as much from my spiritual teachers and the
Divine.

I want to conclude by emphasizing the most important practices
of Soul Mind Body Medicine. I have presented many theories and a
multitude of meditations, exercises, and techniques. They have dealt
not only with health and healing but also with ancient philosophies,
modern scientific insights, soul wisdom, and the spiritual journey. I
trust that by now you understand that all these topics are closely interrelated and that, in particular, the soul is the essence of health and
healing, and also of life.

Before you finish this book, imprint the essence of Soul Mind Body Medicine on your heart and soul. It will help you extract the greatest benefit from this breakthrough healing system. It will serve your healing; bless your life; transform your soul, mind, and body; enlighten your soul; increase your spiritual standing; promote love, peace, and harmony within you and among all souls; and, finally, advance the universe to *Wan Ling Rong He*: all souls joining as one.

Here now is the essence, the *soul*, of Soul Mind Body Medicine.

INNER PEACE

Maintain inner peace all the time. It will put your systems, organs, and cells at peace. Cellular vibration will be smooth and balanced. Energy will flow fluently. Five thousand years ago the Yellow Emperor stated: *Zheng chi cun nei, xie bu xiang gan.* "If you have strong immunity, energy, and vitality, sickness will not come to you."

Inner peace is the key to building strong immunity, increasing energy, and boosting vitality. Keep this wisdom in your mind at all times, and bring inner peace to every aspect of your life. Doing this does require training and practice. Whenever you find yourself irritated or agitated, calm down completely right away and chant *love, peace, and harmony*. Repeat these four words again and again until you return to inner peace. This practice is very simple but very important.

PURIFICATION

We need to purify the soul, mind, and body. Many people attempt to cleanse the body through diet, herbs, exercise, and various treatments. This is important. Many people meditate to purify the mind. This is also important. But how many people know how to purify the soul? How many are even aware of the importance of purifying the soul?

As you now know, purifying the soul is vital. To purify the soul is to cleanse karma, the mistakes one has made in previous lives and in this life. The secret for cleansing karma is to apply forgiveness. In chapter 5, "Universal Meditation," I have shared specific wisdom and practices for offering forgiveness. Apply forgiveness and offer unconditional universal service. This is the golden key to purification, to healing, and to your life and soul journeys. Offer universal love, forgiveness, peace, healing, blessing, harmony, and enlightenment without asking or expecting anything in return.

Giving and sharing are honors. When you offer service to humanity, you may not receive an immediate material or other physical reward, but you will receive great spiritual rewards that you may never consciously realize. You could be spared from a serious car accident, a major illness, a troubled relationship, or a business failure. The Akashic Records note every one of your activities, behaviors, and thoughts. Heaven is the most fair. Offering service will guarantee that you receive the best blessing from the Divine. Although it's an old adage, "giving is receiving" is one of the most important spiritual laws. Purify your soul by offering unconditional universal service.

LOVE AND FORGIVENESS

Love yourself. Love others. Forgive yourself. Forgive others. These are golden keys to healing. From your heart and soul, apply love and forgiveness. For example, if you have back pain, relax completely, and say "hello" to your back: *Dear soul, mind, and body of my back, I love you. Dear the Divine and the universe, if there is any spiritual reason for my backache, please forgive me. Love, peace, healing, harmony. Love, peace, healing, harmony. Love, peace, healing, harmony. Love, peace, healing, harmony.* When you say "love, peace, healing, harmony" to your back, completely open your heart and soul to give love and to receive love from the Divine and the universe. Over the years, I have heard many heart-touching stories from those who have received healing and blessing through love and forgiveness. This is another very simple and practical way to receive healing and blessing power that is beyond comprehension. Continue to give yourself true love for five to ten minutes, and open your heart and soul to receive love from the Divine and the spiritual world. You will hardly believe what life transformation could happen so quickly. Love melts any blockage. Forgiveness brings peace.

3396815 (*SAN SAN JIU LIU BA YAO WU*)

The practice is very simple. Say: *Dear soul, mind, and body of 3396815, I love you, honor you, and appreciate you. Could you help me to heal* _____? *Could you bless my life for* _____? *I'm very grateful. Thank you.* Then you repeat *San San Jiu Liu Ba Yao Wu* for at least five minutes, the longer the better. The number 3396815 is a divine treasure for healing and blessing. Access its power and receive its healing and blessing at any time.

SHA'S GOLDEN HEALING BALL

This is another divine treasure for healing and blessing. You can invoke Sha's Golden Healing Ball anytime, anywhere: *Dear soul, mind, and body of Sha's Golden Healing Ball, I love you, honor you, and appreciate you. Could you come to me to give me a healing and blessing? I'm very grateful. Thank you.* Then, enjoy the power and the blessing of Sha's Golden Healing Ball as you chant *Sha's Golden Healing Ball* or *3396815* for at least five minutes, the longer the better.

UNIVERSAL MEDITATION

Use this breakthrough meditation to boost energy and to heal yourself, your loved ones, society, Mother Earth, and the universe. Use this practice to transform every aspect of your life. You only need one minute to practice effectively. Concentrate and focus fully on love, peace, and harmony for just one minute to apply Universal Meditation in your abdomen. The benefits are waiting for you.

SAY HELLO HEALING AND SAY HELLO BLESSING

This is the simplest and most powerful healing and blessing technique of Soul Mind Body Medicine. In fact, it is the most powerful technique for all spiritual blessings. Although many people know how to say "hello" to saints, Buddhas, healing angels, and the Divine, the results they receive can be quite different. Some people receive a miracle result instantly. Some people get no result at all. Results depend on the following considerations:

- How much bad karma do you have? (Ideally, you are karma free.)

- How much do you want to serve humanity? (The best answer is "unconditionally.")

- How much faith in and loyalty to the spiritual world do you have? (The best answers are "total" and "total.")

- How much of a contribution have you made to the universe? (Ideally, you've made some large ones.)

You can say "hello" to your inner souls — systems, organs, cells, DNA, and RNA. You can also say "hello" to saints, Buddhas, and healing angels in the spiritual world. You can absolutely directly invoke the Divine. Remember, the key spiritual law is that giving is receiving. Giving is unconditional universal service.

❧◎❧

Let me give you one more treasure for prevention now. This practice combines physical actions with visualization.

Sit down properly, with your back straight. Contract your anus a little. Rotate your tongue all around your mouth without allowing it to touch any surface within your mouth. This should produce a steady flow of saliva. When you swallow the saliva, imagine that it goes down your esophagus and through your stomach to your Lower

Dan Tian. Visualize a golden light ball glowing there. When the saliva reaches the golden ball, it turns to steam. The steam ascends through the trunk of your body up to your tongue. This process repeats as you continue the practice for five minutes.

Do this practice a few times a day. Each time, you will receive instant nourishment, boost your energy, gain immunity, prevent sickness, and gain great healing benefits. If you can just sit and do this practice in a deep meditative state for a half hour or longer, the blessing you will receive is beyond comprehension.

This practice exemplifies the statement *Di chi shang sheng, tian chi xia jiang*: "Earth's energy ascends. Heaven's energy descends." *Di* (Earth) is yin. *Tian* (Heaven) is yang. Yin and yang connect with and nourish each other. The saliva produced by rotating the tongue is Heaven's water (*tian chi*). When you swallow this water, *tian chi xia jiang*. When the water reaches your Lower Dan Tian, it transforms to steam (*di chi*). When the steam rises, *di chi shang sheng*.

❧❀❧

It is my honor to close with a final healing and blessing. Follow me:

> *San San Jiu Liu Ba Yao Wu (3396815)*
> *San San Jiu Liu Ba Yao Wu (3396815)*
> *San San Jiu Liu Ba Yao Wu (3396815)*

Dear soul, mind, and body of my systems, organs, cells, DNA, and RNA, I love you, honor you, and appreciate you. You have the power to heal yourselves. Do a good job. Thank you.

Dear soul, mind, and body of the Divine, I love you, honor you, and bow down to you. Could you give me a divine healing and blessing? I'm very grateful. Thank you.

> *San San Jiu Liu Ba Yao Wu (3396815)*
> *San San Jiu Liu Ba Yao Wu (3396815)*
> *San San Jiu Liu Ba Yao Wu (3396815)*

Repeat this divine order as quickly as possible, as many times as you can. In your mind, there are only these thoughts: *I am healed. I am blessed. Illness is prevented. I am protected.*

I send my greatest love and service to each of you. I am a servant to each of you. I am a servant to all humanity. I am a servant to every soul of the universe.

I love my heart and soul.
I love all humanity.
Join hearts and souls together.
Love, peace, and harmony.
Love, peace, and harmony.

Thank you. Thank you. Thank you.

Healing Blessings from My Soul

In *Soul Mind Body Medicine* I have revealed many sacred secrets of soul healing. To conclude this book, I am very honored to offer my soul in service to all humanity and all souls in Jiu Tian (the nine layers of Heaven) and the universe.

To receive my soul healing service, silently say from the bottom of your heart: *Dear soul of Zhi Gang Sha, I love you. Could you give me a soul healing for my* _____ [name the unhealthy conditions for which you would like to receive healing blessings]? *I am grateful. Thank you.* Then, completely relax. Sit up straight or lie down quietly for three minutes. Close your eyes to receive the healing blessings from my soul.

There is no limit to how often you can receive this healing service from my soul. Each time, request and receive for at least three minutes — the longer, the better. When you have concluded receiving the healing blessings, remember to say "thank you" as a spiritual courtesy.

I offer this healing service to you anytime and anywhere on Mother Earth and in the entire universe. I open my soul to offer this

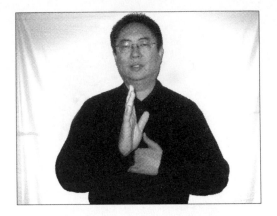

Figure 43. *Healing blessings from my soul*

because I am an unconditional universal servant. I am offering universal service, which includes universal love, forgiveness, peace, healing, blessing, harmony, and enlightenment. May my soul serve you well.

There is another way to receive my soul healing. Look at my picture above and silently say from the bottom of your heart: *Dear soul of Zhi Gang Sha, I love you. Could you give me a soul healing for my* _____ [name the unhealthy conditions for which you would like to receive healing blessings]? *I am grateful. Thank you.* Then, completely relax. Sit up straight or lie down quietly and continue to look at my picture for three minutes to receive healing blessings from my soul.

As a universal healer and servant, I am very blessed to have been given the divine honor and privilege of transmitting divine healing and blessing treasures to humanity. These treasures include Soul Software, Soul Herbs, Soul Healing Water, Soul Acupuncture, Soul Food, Soul Rainbow Light Ball and Soul Rainbow Liquid Spring, Soul Operation, and Soul Transplant. Recipients can invoke these permanent divine treasures anytime and anywhere to receive divine healing and blessing. I am extremely honored to be a universal servant.

Thank you. Thank you. Thank you.

Acknowledgments

I deeply appreciate all my teachers of tai chi, qi gong, kung fu, I Ching, and feng shui. Their teaching has given me a deep knowledge of these ancient Chinese arts. Without their teaching, I could not have written this book as well.

I deeply appreciate my teachers of Buddhism, Taoism, and Confucianism. The wisdom of these three Chinese cultural treasures has nourished me and helped develop my spiritual wisdom, knowledge, and practice. Without their teaching, I couldn't have written this book as well.

I deeply appreciate my teachers of Western and traditional Chinese medicine. They taught me the wisdom of medicine. Without their teaching, I couldn't have written this book as well.

I deeply appreciate my most beloved spiritual father, Dr. Zhi Chen Guo. He taught me the secret wisdom, knowledge, and practice of energy healing, spiritual healing, and developing the intelligence and power of the mind and soul. Without his teaching, it would have been impossible to write this book. I thank Master Guo from the bottom of my heart.

I deeply appreciate Dr. John Gray for his great guidance in my writing and teaching and for his incredible support of my journey to the United States; Dr. and Reverend Michael Beckwith for his tremendous support of my journey; and Dr. Wayne Dyer, Dr. Larry Dossey, Dr. Masaru Emoto, Marianne Williamson, and Debbie Ford for their endorsement and great support of my work.

I deeply appreciate Diana Gold Holland for writing a marvelous and powerful proposal for this book, May Guey Chew for her careful and thoughtful initial editing of two chapters to support the book proposal, and Kara M. Jewell for supporting the editing and being a key assistant in compiling the photographs. I deeply appreciate Mike Lee of MotoPhoto for his clear and efficient photography. I deeply appreciate Tony Edelstein, Karen Kane, and Mary Ann Casler for the cover design.

I deeply appreciate eleven divine communicators, of the many I have trained, for their divine flow, which gave me further guidance on the book and the book cover: Marilyn Smith, Anita Eubank, Millie Luong, Joyce Brown, Patricia Smith, Aubrey Degnan, Patty Baker, Artemas Yaffe, Sandra Sharpe, and Allan Chuck.

I deeply appreciate Millie Luong, general manager of the Institute of Soul Mind Body Medicine, for her great contributions to my mission. I thank my other business leaders, Allan Chuck, Ximena Gavino, and Stan Turczyniak for their contributions. I deeply thank all my business team members, previous and current, for their great contributions. I deeply thank Dr. Peter Hudoba, chairman of the board of Sha Research Foundation, and other members of the Research Foundation for their great contributions. I deeply thank my seven Assistant Teachers, Allan Chuck, Marilyn Smith, Peter Hudoba, Patricia Smith, Aubrey Degnan, Anita Eubank, and Shu Chin Hsu for their great contributions. I deeply thank the hundreds of divine healers and the eighty divine writers whom I have trained for their great contributions to my mission.

I deeply appreciate Allan Chuck for his editing, including the final editing of this book. He synthesized all the wisdom, knowledge, and practice so well. Without his effort, this book could not be in its current shape. I cannot thank Allan enough for his great support of my work and for his wonderful contributions.

I deeply appreciate my publisher, Marc Allen of New World Library, for his care and his great support of my work. I deeply appreciate New World Library's editorial director, Georgia Hughes, for her efficient communication, suggestions, and support. I deeply appreciate New World Library's manuscript editor, Mimi Kusch, for her valuable suggestions for improving the organization and clarity of this book. I deeply appreciate Kristen Cashman, New World Library's managing editor, for coordinating and directing the editorial process. I deeply appreciate Tona Pearce Myers for her expert typesetting of this book. I deeply appreciate Kim Corbin, New World Library's Publicist, and Munro Magruder, New World Library's Marketing Director, for their enthusiastic support of my work.

Last, but hardly least, I thank my parents, wife, and children for their great support of my work and for their great love.

Notes

CHAPTER 2. SOUL OVER MATTER

1. See also my previously published book *Soul Study: A Guide to Accessing Your Highest Powers* (Vancouver: Zhi Neng Press, 1997).
2. See chapter 8, and also consult my books *Power Healing: The Four Keys to Energizing Your Body, Mind & Spirit* (San Francisco: HarperCollins, 2002) and *Zhi Neng Medicine: Revolutionary Self-Healing Methods from China* (Vancouver, BC: Zhi Neng Press, 1996) for more details.

CHAPTER 3. MIND OVER MATTER

1. Zhi Gang Sha, *Power Healing: The Four Keys to Energizing Your Body, Mind & Spirit* (San Francisco: HarperCollins, 2002).

CHAPTER 4. ONE-MINUTE HEALING

1. The special number sequence and mantra, 3396815, can actually be chanted in any language. Benefits will still accrue because of the message, or soul, of this sacred mantra. However, chanting *San San Jiu Liu Ba Yao Wu* in Chinese carries the added benefits of the physical vibration stimulated by the individual Chinese sounds. It is like giving the body an inner massage in a healthy vibrational pattern.

2. For more on this topic, see my book *Sha's Golden Healing Ball: The Perfect Gift* (Vancouver, BC: Zhi Neng Press, 1997), 4–5.

CHAPTER 6. APPLICATIONS OF SOUL MIND BODY MEDICINE

1. Zhi Gang Sha, *Power Healing: The Four Keys to Energizing Your Body, Mind & Spirit* (San Francisco: HarperCollins, 2002).

Index

About the Author

An MD in China and a doctor of traditional Chinese medicine in China and Canada, Dr. Zhi Gang Sha is a master healer and master teacher of healing and spiritual wisdom, knowledge, and practice. Since 2003 he has been a divine direct channel, transmitting hundreds of thousands of divine healing and blessing treasures to humanity.

Sha completed his medical education at Xi'an Jiaotong University and earned a master's degree in Hospital Administration at the University of the Philippines. By the age of twenty, he had already created a unique and powerful form of acupuncture. Sha's acupuncture uses rapid insertion and removal of the needle on only twelve key acupuncture points and incorporates energy and soul healing. Its effectiveness led Sha to be invited by the World Health Organization's International Acupuncture Training Center in Beijing to teach acupuncture and qi gong to foreign physicians.

Since meeting his most revered teacher and master, Dr. Zhi Chen Guo, in 1993, Sha has been committed to his journey of energy healing, spiritual healing, and spiritual teaching, and specifically to his three life missions described in the preface to this book. His journey expanded greatly when he began to write and teach in the United States in earnest in 2000, publishing his pioneering book on self-healing, *Power Healing: The Four Keys to Energizing Your Body, Mind & Spirit* (San Francisco: HarperCollins, 2002). Sha had previously published *Zhi Neng Medicine: Revolutionary Self-Healing Methods from China, Soul Study: A Guide to Accessing Your Highest Powers, Sha's Golden Healing Ball: The Perfect Gift,* and (in Chinese) *Zhi Neng Healing: Illustrated Self-Healing Hand Positions.*

Dr. Sha has been a speaker at the Omega Institute, The Crossings, the Esalen Institute, the Institute of Noetic Sciences, the Agape International Spiritual Center, the second, fourth, and fifth World Congresses on Qigong, the 30th Anniversary SSF-IIIHS International Conference, the Aspen Center for Integrative Health, the Genesys Regional Medical Center, the Learning Annex, the third Annual Integrative Medicine Forum of the University of California at San Francisco, the twelfth International Conference on Anti-Aging and Biotechnologies, the California Institute for Integral Studies, the Integrative Medicine Clinic of Santa Rosa, and the Institute for Transpersonal Psychology.

Named Qigong Master of the Year at the fifth World Congress on Qigong in 2002, Sha has been featured in two PBS documentaries, *Qigong: Ancient Chinese Healing for the 21st Century* and *Power Healing with Master Sha,* on Canadian Learning Television's Power Healing with Master Sha, as well as internationally on television, radio, the Internet, and in print media. The founder of the Institute of Soul Mind Body Medicine, the International Institute of Zhi Neng Medicine, and Sha Research Foundation, Dr. Sha resides in Canada.

Visit www.drsha.com for more information. Contact him at drsha@drsha.com or 1-888-3396815 (toll-free in the U. S. and Canada) if you are interested in having Dr. Sha speak and teach in your area.